SAVE

$5000 FOR GLASSES,
$2500 FOR TOOTHACHE,
AND **$4500** FOR TINNITUS

SAVE

$5000 FOR GLASSES, $2500 FOR TOOTHACHE, AND $4500 FOR TINNITUS

BY LICENSED ACUPUNCTURIST
CHAN HUR

authorHOUSE®

AuthorHouse™
1663 Liberty Drive
Bloomington, IN 47403
www.authorhouse.com
Phone: 1-800-839-8640

Published by AuthorHouse   01/11/2013

ISBN: 978-1-4772-1765-8 (sc)
ISBN: 978-1-4772-1764-1 (e)

Library of Congress Control Number: 2012910342

INTRODUCTION

Everyone understands when we get older, eye vision becomes blurry and dim sighted. I noticed my vision becomes dimmed when I read newspaper. It was more difficult to read small letters. Sometimes I couldn't focus well and hold papers far away back and force, but in vain. I try to avoid reading small letters. This makes me not to read comics which was written with small letters. This made me a little depressed day by day.

When my wife started wearing glasses, I felt sorry for her. She didn't wear glasses when she married to me. This means she got older and felt time really flies. Since then she looked for glasses everyday without an exception. Looking for glasses must be bothersome. When she looked, I joked that you can't find glasses without glasses. I told her and complained that if you put glasses on fixed place, you don't have to look for everyday. When time passed by, she used a large magnifier to read in addition of glasses. When I asked her to get new glasses, she told me insurance covers only every two years, so she was better off to wait a few more months.

I also noticed reading on dark place is more difficult and tried to read later. I then missed reading completely as I didn't read on time and forgot about it. When I have to read with a magnifier as it is absolutely necessary, the magnifier is disappeared as my wife used it and put it somewhere I don't put. I noticed myself being angry once in a while. I argued with my wife that she had to use her own. Sometimes looking for a magnifier takes a time, and couldn't find it.

I saw TV ads saying Lasik surgery enables to see without glasses in 1997. This may be a cool idea and went to the eye doctor. After he examined my eyes, I need glasses and I am not a candidate of Lasik surgery. As I get older, my eye muscle becomes weak, therefore he prescribed eyeglasses. I kept the prescription into my wallet and walked out the room. The corridor was very long. While I walked through the corridor, one word was kept on bothering me that I am getting older. I am only 50 now and can't believe I get older.

Couple of days passed by and one idea came into my mind that I should start an eye exercise. I heard and learned this from my mother, but never practiced since I knew. I determined to practice everyday as I believe it is never late. I did only on around eyes, but I noticed my vision improving after a few years. I can read dictionary's small letters when I read on bright sunny day.

I had a weird experience in 2002. While I walked into the bedroom, I saw sudden green light just like glowfly. I thought it was a lightening bug, but it was not a bug. It was from my eyes. I involved very much in church activity, so I thought I received Holy Spirit. I told my wife next morning I received Holy Spirit. After listening me, she knew something happened to me, but she didn't understand exactly as she didn't experience anything like that. I drove the car a few days later and saw some kind of spider web from my eyes. Now I knew that I didn't receive Holy Spirit, but something wrong with my eyes. I went to the same eye doctor. After he examined, it is a floater that came out of eyeball. Depending on angle, it may look like spider web, flying fly or glowfly. Doctor advised me that I have to come and see him every month as this may be a dangerous sign. I asked him what I or he can do. Doctor said nothing. I didn't go to see him as I believe he wanted to make money on me. He looked my chart for the previous one and new one alternately a few times and said my vision was improved than 5 years ago. Is that normal when we get older our vision dimmer? In my case it was a reverse.

My wife saw what I am doing. She learned from me and started practicing. I don't remember exactly when, but she didn't use wide magnifier anymore, even though she still wears glasses.

Everyone understands wearing glasses is bothersome. There are limited ways not to wear glasses. What about contact lenses? This may look natural as a person doesn't wear glasses, however contact lenses may cause bad for eyes in my opinion. Here is why. Body heat is supposed to rise. When heat rises, it is shown with many different ways: sweating or breathing. All heat is supposed to rise to head. When young person has heat from stomach, it rises into face and can't be released, this shows as pimples. When heat rises, some of them may come out from mouth and some comes out from the nose. Whatever remained heat will reach into eyes, heat is supposed to be released through eyes. When heat reaches to contact lenses, how is the heat able to be released? This will block heat resulting on pupils. Many believe that improper cleansing or wearing them during sleep cause keratitis. I believe this statement, but also by blockage from heat releasing. I heard once keratitis is caused 35% by contact lenses.

Reason for bad vision

Bad vision comes from poor nutrition and oxygen supply into eyes. There are no good reasons to be explained without poor nutrition and oxygen. The only answer should be proper blood circulation is mandatory. There are a few ways to improve for better blood circulation such as exercise, bath, small amount of alcohol, and spicy foods and etc.

Some with poor blood circulation have cold constitution. Making body warm helps not only for general health, but also bad vision.

Some have hot constitution. Hotness means producing more heat than normal. Heat usually consumes moisture resulting in eye dryness. Removing extra heat is the answer in this case. This can be achieved by herb and acupuncture. I suggest drinking a tea like Ji Meng tea listed in this book.

Everyone knows exercise is good, but practicing is another matter. It is difficult to spare the time for that. There is someone who has no energy to exercise on the worst case.

Alcohol, spicy foods and exercising are caused sweating sometimes. These raise body heat helping better blood circulation. I suggest little amount of sweating is good, but excessive sweating is not good. In my opinion, it is better off sweating in 5 minutes. We must be careful that spicy foods may cause irritation against weak stomach. Even though alcohol is good originally, drinking more than supposed to be means worse than no drinking.

All the above methods are good for general health, but not for specific organs. Certain exercise may help specific organ or body. Learning these kinds of exercises may be difficult and takes a lot of time. However doing all these will benefit you and help for your health.

One of good ways is acupuncture treatments. Acupuncture theory explains eyes are closely related with liver. This means treating liver helps better blood circulation and better vision. As liver has a function of detoxication, acupuncture treatment may relieve toxics accumulated in the liver. I heard many times as soon as I tap needles, patients shout my vision becomes brighter instantly. Acupuncture text books explain that 5 zang organs are related with eyeballs. This means treating all 5 zang organs are expected for better results. 5zangs mean liver, heart, spleen (pancreas), lung and kidney.

Cataract and Glaucoma

I have patients one in a while that they had an eye surgery before and the same problem occurred. The reason is very simple to me. The surgery was only for symptom and the real cause was not solved.

What is the real cause?

Cataract usually happens to lung weakness. Glaucoma happens to liver related. This is based on acupuncture theory and my experience. If anyone has cataract or glaucoma, please consider seeing acupuncturist.

Other ways many people practice

1. Young students in China learn and practice in the elementary school. There are couple of ways. One method that my patient showed me was using second knuckle of second finger. Press the inner eye and slide it out to outer eye. I believe this is unique that no other school does as far as I know.

2. When you rub palms, this creates heat. Put both palms cover eyes. You have to hold tight

with fingers. This is not recommended for person with hot constitution.

3. Meditation. You try to receive universe energy through vertex of head and send to eyes.

4. Put small letters on the wall. Try to concentrate for reading from certain distance. When you are able to read, you move a little further out from the original point. One thing careful is not to winking as far as you can.

5. Move eyes from up to bottom, bottom to up, left to right, right to left, diagonally up and down. Make circles with eyes by clockwise and counter clockwise. I suggest you do this exercise when you are alone. If someone looks at you, you may look like suffering with epilepsy.

All above would help you, but this will take your time except 1 and 2.

Now you can practice my way and discover how effective and easy as soon as you memorize it in order.

Challenge for Dementia Etc. beyond Eye Vision

When we get older, we tent to forget easily. We experience once in a while that we went another room to do or find something, then forgot totally what to do and don't know why we are here. I don't have a talent to memorize person's name since childhood. I gave up memorizing names long time ago.

Some idea came to my mind while I do eye exercising, what about to expend to face and head. If I add acupressure theory or massage on face and head and shoulder, it may do great impact on them. Western medicine believes brain memory is based on brain. If this idea is right and we stimulate all acupuncture points on head, the following exercise is going to help to improve memory

Method to
Practice Regularly

Everyone has limited 24 hours a day. There is no discrimination between rich or poor, man or woman, young or old, and smart or stupid. I believe how to utilize our time well makes our life different.

Most of us go to bathroom for bowel movement once a day. Some goes every 2 or 3 days. This is a kind of constipation in my standard, as someone claims that is normal. I suggest changing daily habit, taking more fibers and acupuncture treatments. Try jumping rope. This will help for peristaltic movement of large intestine.

Let me introduce what I do. I do bowel movement, eye exercise, and reading Bible at the same time. When I sit on the toilet bowl, I open my Bible which is located on the top of water tank. When I read one page on Bible, I do one group which will be explained shortly.

I thought in the beginning reading Bible during bowel movement was unrespectable for God. I know myself as soon as I get out of the bathroom, I don't try to find a time to sit down and read Bible. I also realize that God creates me to do the bowel movement. I concluded reading Bible in this way is better than not reading. If you are not a Christian, you can read your Holy books, books or even newspapers. There is no limitation.

Someone doesn't stay in the bathroom for a long time. This person can read half page or even quarter page on each group.

Concern about that sitting long on toilet bowl causes hemorrhoids
This sounds right and may be true. The true reason for hemorrhoids is due to constipation on most cases. Pushing hard downwards is the problem. Another is due to spleen qi deficiency. Constipation or spleen qi deficiency is real health issue. It is better off to get proper treatment. You don't have to worry about

hemorrhoids if bowel movement is normal even though you sit for a long sitting.

Do you believe that sitting on chair for a long time causes hemorrhoids? What about with bicycle or horse riding? This may be possible, but I don't' believe 5-20 minutes a day would be a problem for that.

There are many good reasons if you stay long at toilet bowl. You can read more books. Believe me that you can study better sometimes as no one bothers you. There is a good chance that you eliminate all feces. Is there any good reason to carry any unnecessary feces?

How long do we have this exercise?
Doing more is better. But we all have busy life. Doing only this exercise is impossible.

I read Bible 14 pages a day. I don't suggest this to everyone. This takes a time usually a little over 20 minutes. I suggest one minute per group or 30 seconds per group depending on your preference. The important thing is you practice every day.

Please note that you may feel better on certain group than another group. If you have a better feeling, you do this part longer.

How long does this exercise make effectiveness?

It depends on individuals. Some experience immediately saying "Hey, I can read the name on business card." Some say like me that it may be possible to read newspaper without a difficulty. Generally speaking it will take 6 to 9 months if you continue to work on. Please note that Group 10 can be done anytime. You also press acupuncture points listed in this book any times, too.

Can you do this anytime?

Yes, you can do anytime. You must do this exercise especially when eyes become tired after reading a book, or spending long time in front of computer. Most important thing is exercising regularly every day.

One more important thing is to press more on the weak area. Weak points mean experiencing more pain and making us feel good.

When you press ST 1, it may make you feel better than UB 1. This means ST 1 point is weaker than UB 1.

When you have gum pain, you press gum more than other area. This helps better blood circulation.

When eyes become tired

1. Try to look outside through windows

   Green leaves, or trees or especially blue sky are very good. Some try to look TV or read newspaper, but this makes worse, not recommended at all.

2. Food selection based on individual constitution

   It is important to take better foods based on for individual constitution. When eyes become dimmer, it is more important to choose better foods for individuals.

3. We understand that we should take a break while on working. I suggest taking a break of 10 minutes after 50 minutes of working.

4. When we get older, it is quite natural that eyes vision becomes bad. In order not to make eyes tired, try to read with large size of letter with computer. If there is large type of books available, choose large type book. For example, there are many sizes of printed books on Bible.

Eye Exercise PLUS

While I do eye exercising, I believe I can improve and expend this exercising into not only for eye, but also face, head and shoulder. This is based on acupuncture theory. Most acupuncture points are covered here with a few exceptions. Many are added even though these are regular points, but very helpful for me. If you continue this exercising, you can expect the followings.

Digestion improvement

Rhinitis

Allergy

Gum disease

Tinnitus

Difficult hearing

Headache

Wrinkle removal

Dementia

I just name a few, however you can expect any symptoms related with head, such as eyes, nose, mouth, and ears.

My hope

I have practiced since 1997. It is now 2012, so almost 14 years. If I wear glasses, there was a good chance I may switch glasses every two years as the insurance company covers every two years. Insurance companies cover only limited portion. They don't cover 100% for glasses. Good glasses may be over $700-800. This means I save more than $5000 for glasses.

I hope I want to live up to 140 years old, even though life is depending on God. I hope I don't wear glasses until I die. If so, my hope may be too extreme. I hope I don't wear glasses another 14-16 years until I am 80 years old.

Another hope
All insurance companies buy this book and provide all their policy holders. If everyone follows, insurance company will pay less as policy holders become healthy and there is no need to claim lots of money.

Group 1

Use second finger to fifth finger. Press from under diaphragmatic to pubic. When you feel some kind of pain or lump, you press hard and longer. If possible, it is better from the top to downward.

If anyone have digestion problem, follow this. Transverse colon that is located around umbilicus is pressed from right to left. If there is stomach or small intestine problem, press stomach from left to right. The reason is stomach is connected into duodenum. Duodenum is located on right side. Small intestine connects to ascending large intestine on right side.

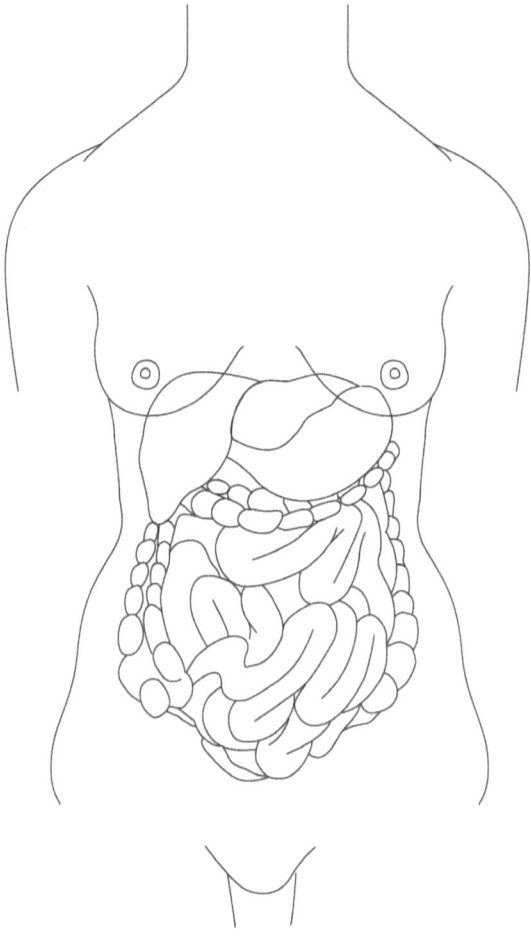

Group 1

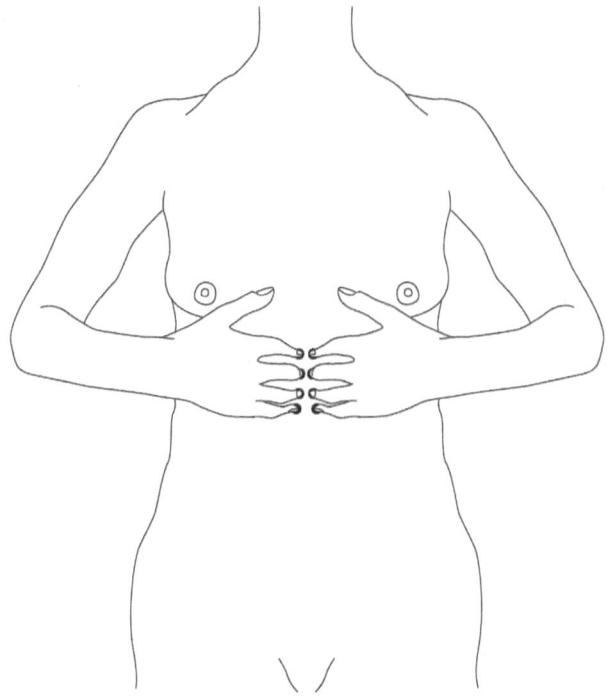

Group 1

Group 2

A. Press thumb into UB1[1]. Simultaneously try to rub UB2[2] with index finger knuckles from inner area to outwards. This way makes Yintang[3] less wrinkle.

B. Press pinky fingers into UB2 area of the eyebrows, while index fingers press into UB3[4], inside hairline.

UB1:   in the depression slightly above the inner canthus
UB2:   on the medial extremity of the eyebrow
Yintang: midway between the medial ends of the two eyebrows
UB3:   directly above the medial end of the eyebrow

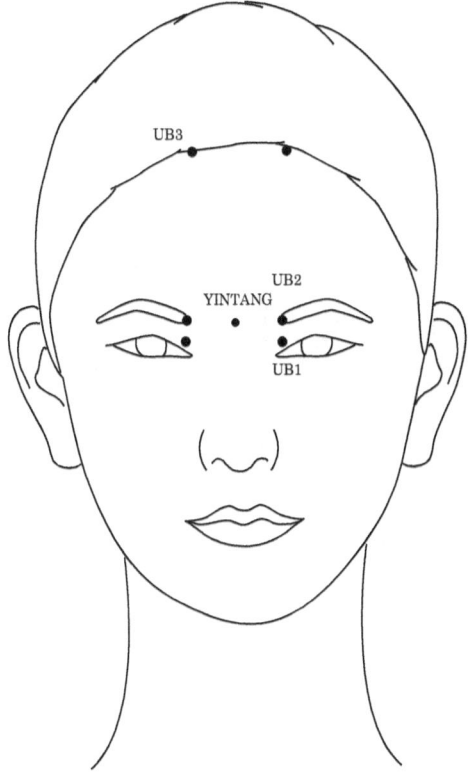

Group 2

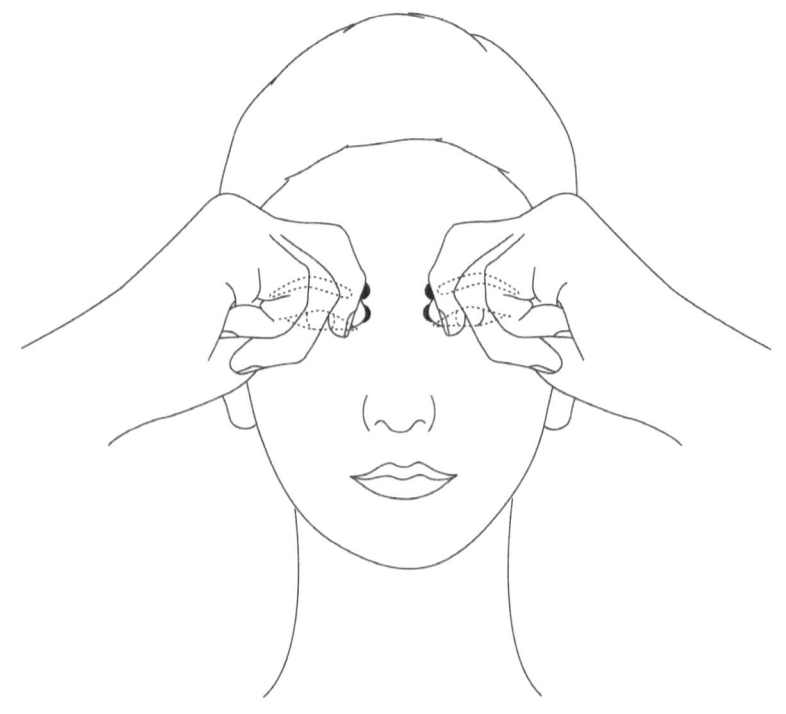

Group 2-A

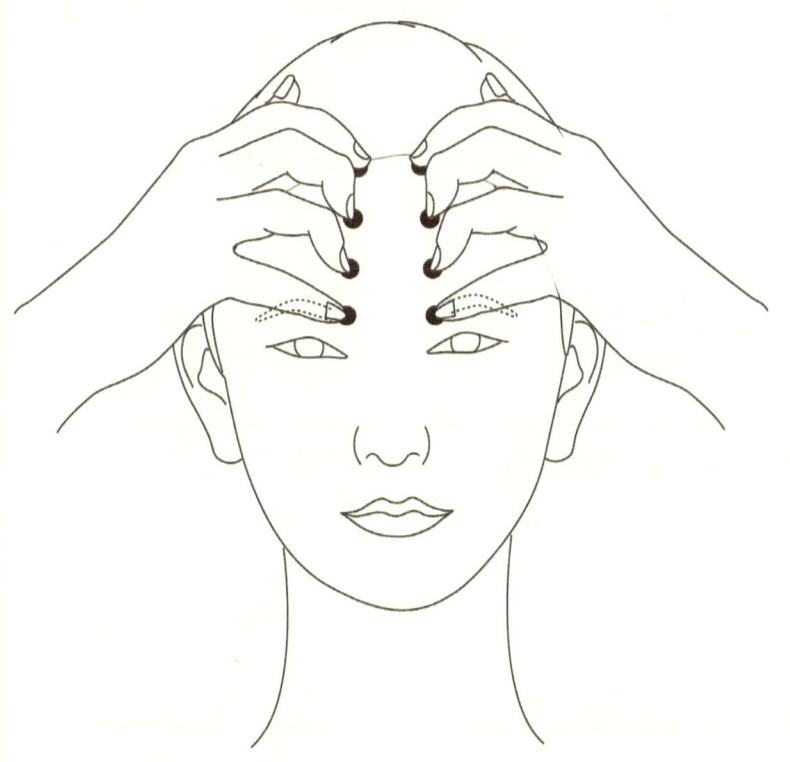

Group 2-B

Group 3

Index fingers press under the eyes into ST1[5], while the thumbs massage along the upper gum. Pinky fingers massage and press into the center of the upper gum line.

- You can't do all upper gum with this. You can use tips under Group 12.

A solution for some very expensive dental expenses

Sterilize a needle with alcohol. Find the painful or swollen area. Inject a needle into the painful area in about 3-5 spots. Close the mouth and try to suck blood out. Spit out blood. Repeat this procedure until no more blood comes out. You might worry that needle insertion would be painful. Yes, but less painful than an anesthesia injection by a dentist. You can avoid this anesthesia injection from the dentist anyhow.

ST1:   directly below the pupil, between the eyeball and the infraorbital ridge

Prevent infection. Dentists prescribe drugs to prevent infection. If you can't go to a dentist, you can't have drugs. Buy bamboo salt. This is sold in Korean supermarket. Make a solution of 0.9%. If you can't find bamboo salt, try sea salt instead. Rinse mouth with this solution often, especially after meals. I never heard of any infection with this method but continue to monitor your tooth for infection.

Toothache is the just a manifestation of organs' problems. Kidney governs bone according to TCM. There are a lot of issues to discuss, but this is too technical for ordinary patients.

Even though you get a new tooth or bridge, stagnation or stasis remains the same around tooth and gum. These must be removed in order to prevent further damage. It is very necessary to have better blood circulation around problem teeth. To prevent further worse developments, go and see an acupuncturist who understands this concept.

One patient mentioned toothache. I explained this method and he went home and did exactly what I told him. Next morning he found no pain at all. He called his dentist to cancel the appointment. When he returned to me, he told me he saved $2500 for his dental bill.

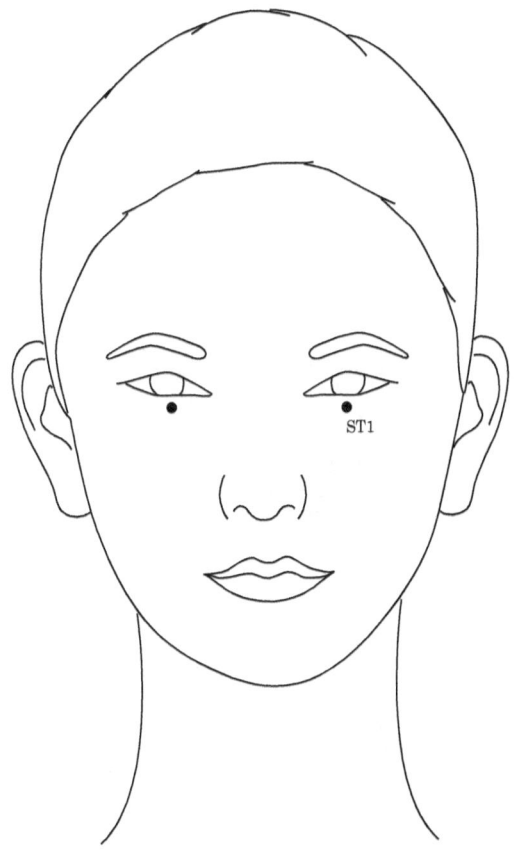

ST1

Group 3

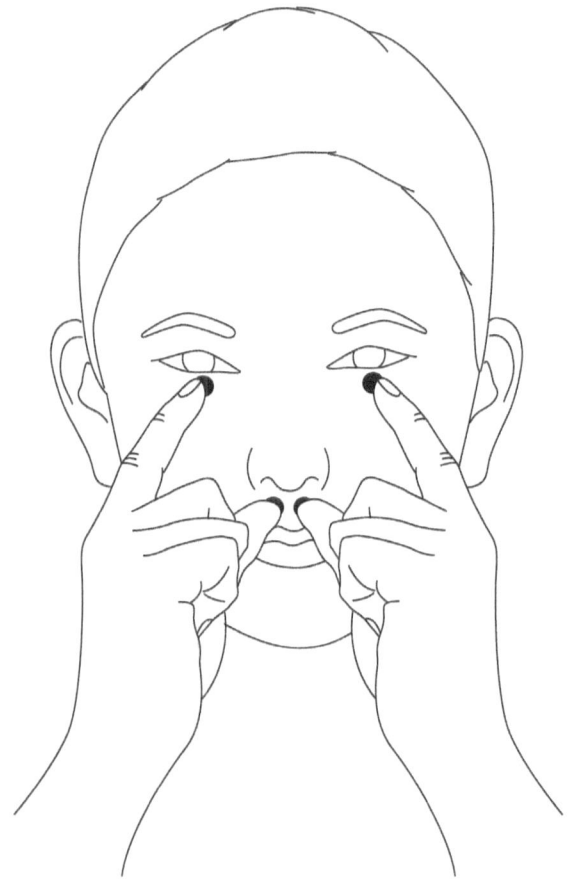

Group 3-A

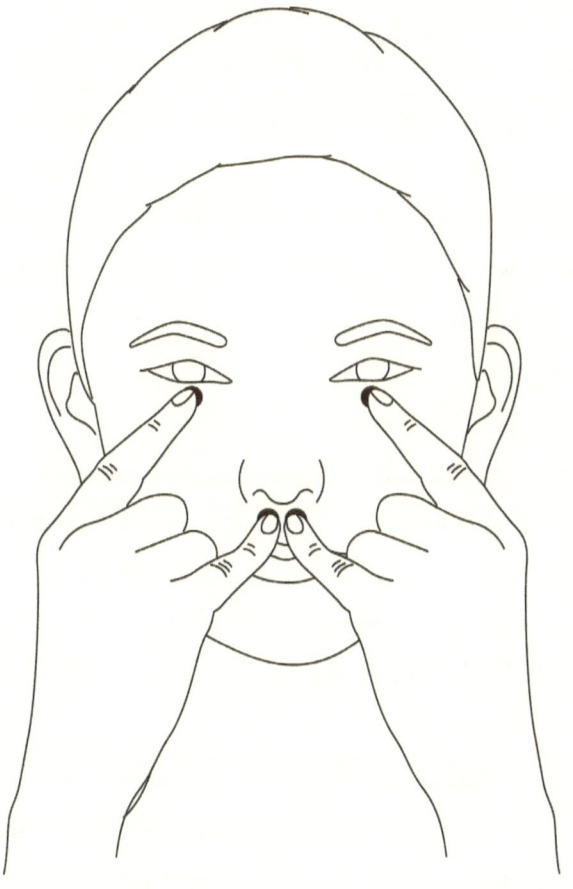

Group 3-B

Dental Implants

When I went to the dentist for a loose bridge, my dentist suggested tooth implants. A tooth (dental) implant is an artificial tooth root placed in your jaw to hold a replacement tooth or bridge. He explained how to make a tooth implant, which is to make a hole into the bone and set up a new screw and build up a new tooth. It was a cool idea. However I told my dentist I wouldn't do that as I am an acupuncturist. He asked me why.

I answered that all bones contain nerves and bone marrow. As soon as you make a hole into bones, even normal healthy bone will start to deteriorate. There are invisible routes to nourish bones for nerves and bone marrow. These routes will be destroyed or blocked by making holes.

My dentist told me that an implant makes bone strong. Do you agree with that? In my opinion this dentist may make more money from implanting than a denture. An implant is a lot more expensive than a removable denture, even though implant price has come down a lot now than when first introduced. I personally prefer a denture, which is a great invention, even though biting ability is far less than implant. When we get older, it is not desirable anyhow to bite or chew hard food for good digestion. The reason I choose denture is not because of steep price.

According to acupuncture theory bones are governed by kidney. Teeth also belong to bone. When teeth have problems, we may say these ultimately come from kidney dysfunction. On the top of that, making a hole into bone may cause further damage against kidney. Acupuncturists are very careful not to touch bone with acupuncture needles when tapping. Touching bone with a needle means maybe poking kidney with a needle in theory. If this theory is right, what about making a hole with a drill? Some dentists claim that striking upper and lower teeth together is good for preventing dementia. Teeth implant would satisfy this purpose. It is true, however there are another ways to achieve this by facial or eye exercise.

How to care for your dental implant already done?
You paid lots of money for a tooth implant. It is an expensive one; therefore you have to keep it well

always. Otherwise it will cost you more money and inconvenience and suffering. The answer how to avoid losing the implant is to strengthen the bone that is holding the implant by activating better blood circulation around related bone. Without proper nutrition on bone, there is a good chance for bone to be withered. This withering process will make implant loose. It is very necessary to get regular checkups twice a year to maintain the implant.

In addition it would be very good idea to use acupuncture for good bone maintenance. As there is no nerve in implant, you may feel no pain even though the bone has a problem. It may be too late when you notice inflammation on gum or bone. Acupuncture treatments will prevent inflammation on gum around implant area, and also prevent bone withering causing loose screwing. This acupuncture treatment is the least expensive way to maintain healthy implant.

Group 4

Index fingers press under Quihou[6], slightly outside of center, as thumbs press sequentially near the cheekbone from ST5[7], SI 18[8], and ST7[9] to GB3[10].

QIUHOU: at the junction of the lateral ¼ and the medial ¾ of the infraorbital margin

ST5: anterior to the angle of mandible, on the anterior border of the attached portion of muscle masseter, where the pulsation of the facial artery is palpable, in the groove-like depression appearing when the cheek is bulged

SI18: directly below the outer canthus, in the depression on the lower border of zygoma

ST7: on the face anterior to the ear, in the depression between the zygomatic arch and mandibular notch. This point is located with the mouth closed.

GB3: in the front of the ear, on the upper border of the zygomatic arch, in the depression directly above ST7

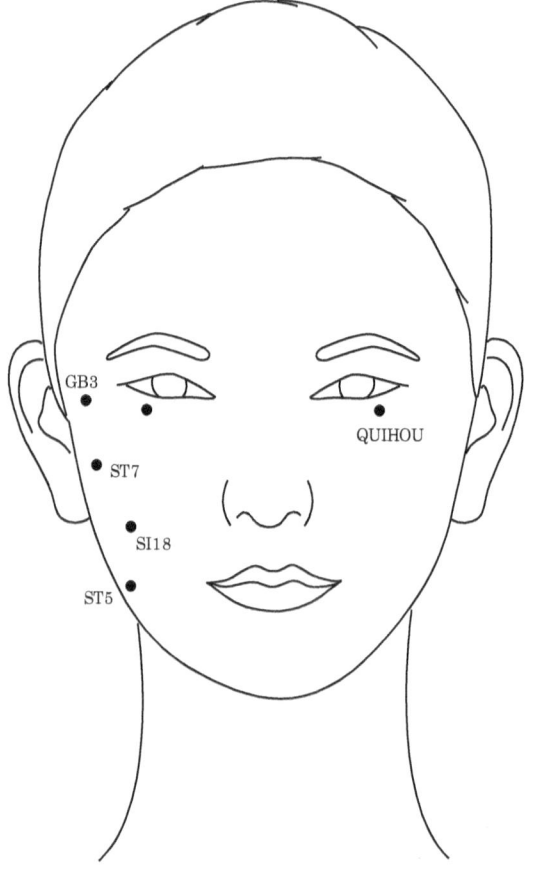

Group 4

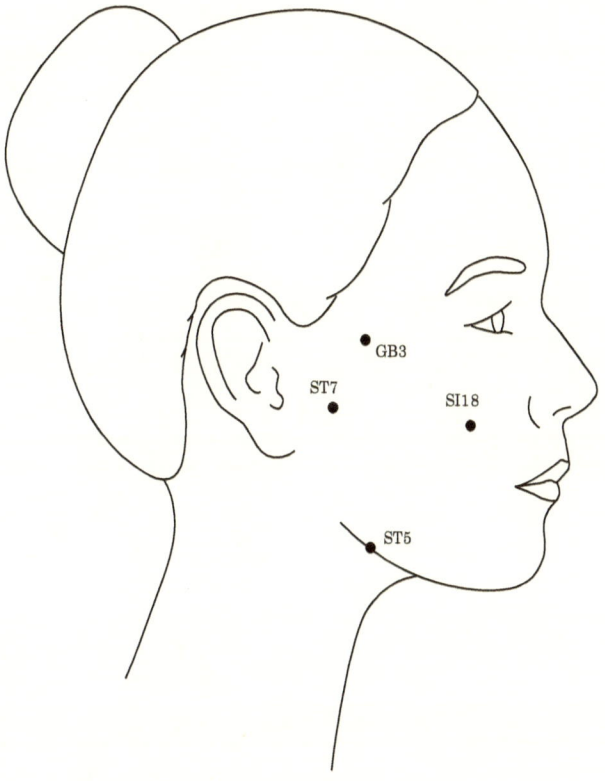

Group 4

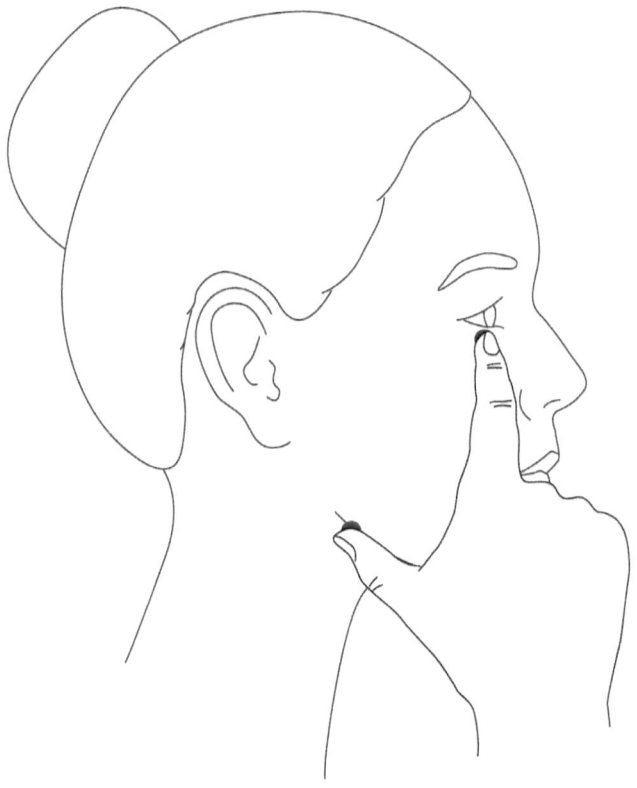

Group 4-ST5

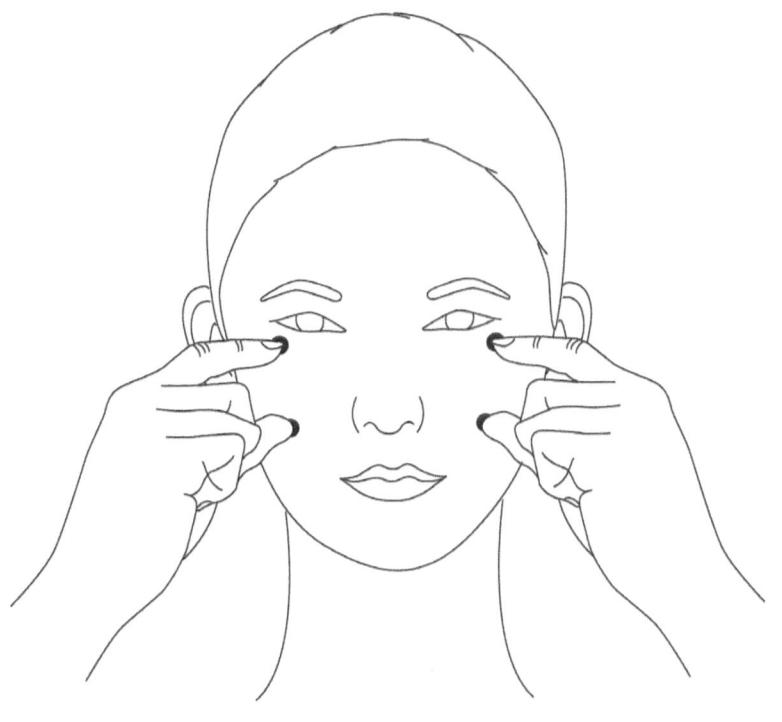

Group 4-SI18

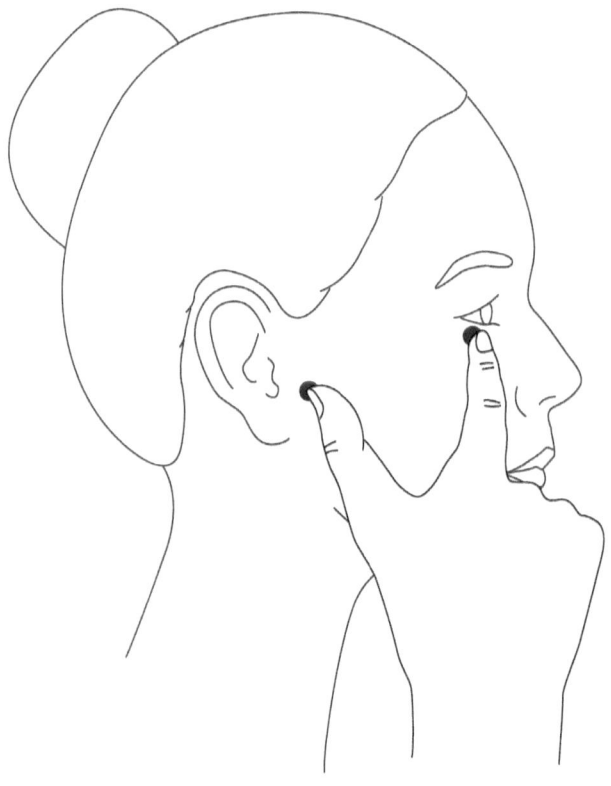

Group 4-ST7

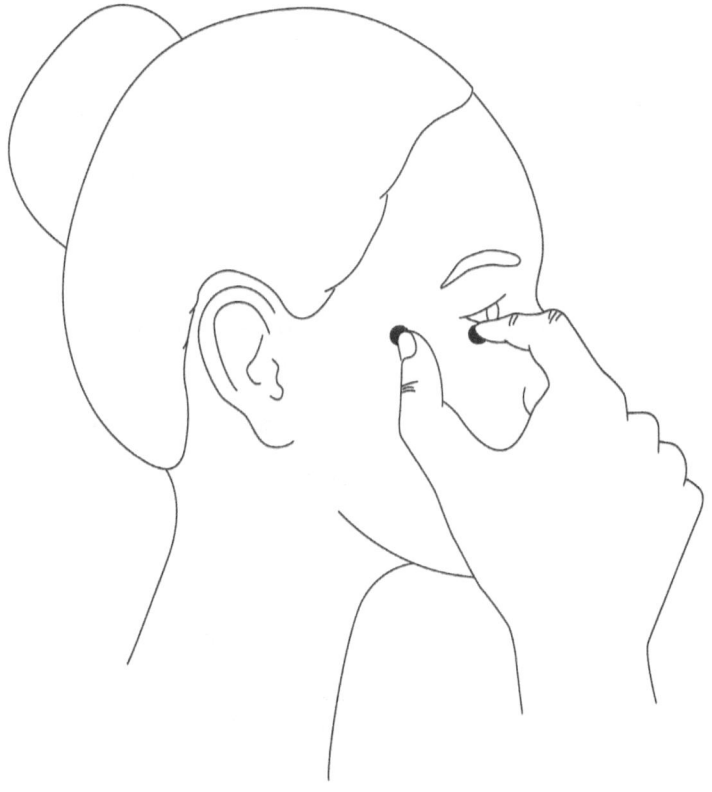

Group 4-GB3

Group 5

A. Forefingers[11] press GB1 into the outside the corners of the eyes, as thumbs press into the points GB2[12], SI 19[13], SJ21[14] near the ears.

B. Thumbs press into the upper sides of eyes, SJ20, as third and fourth fingers massage from the beginning of eyebrow to the end of eyebrow.

C. Move and press thumbs into the points between SJ20 and Taiyang, as second, third and fourth fingers collected together massage from the middle of eyebrows into inside hairline, GB14[15].

GB1:   0.5 cun lateral to the outer canthus, in the depression on the lateral side of the orbit
Cun means about ¾ inch depending on person.

GB2:   anterior to the intertragic notch, at the posterior bordor of the condyloid process of the mandible. The point is located with the mouth open.

SI19:   anterior to the tragus and posterior to the condyloid process of the mandible, in the depression formed when the mouth is open.

SJ21:   in the depression anterior to the supratragic notch and slightly superior to the condyloid process of the mandible. The point is located with mouth open.

GB14:   on the forehead, directly above the pupil, 1 cun directly above the midpoint of the eyebrow

Yuyao: at the midpoint of the eyebrow, directly above the pupil

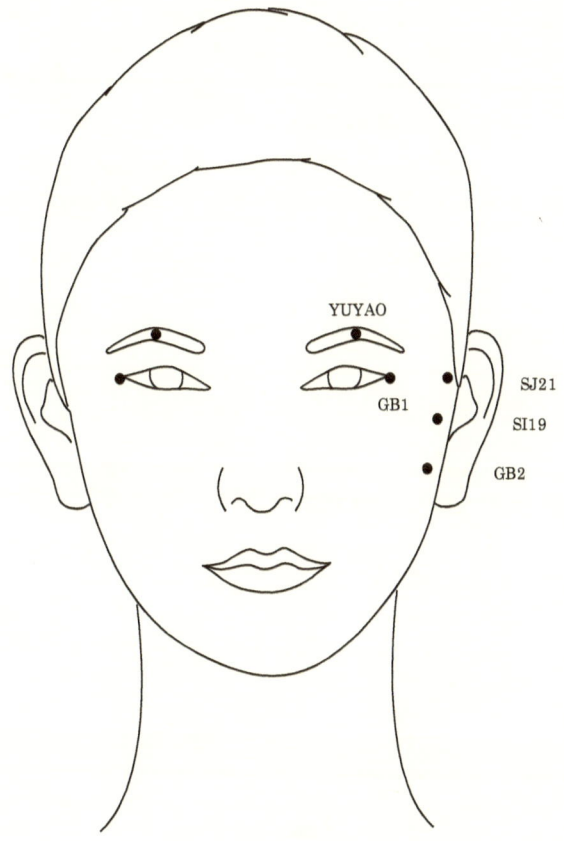

YUYAO

GB1

SJ21

SI19

GB2

Group 5

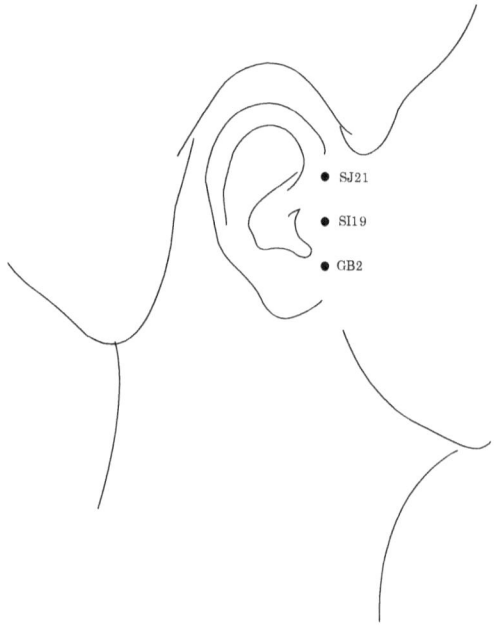

Group 5-A

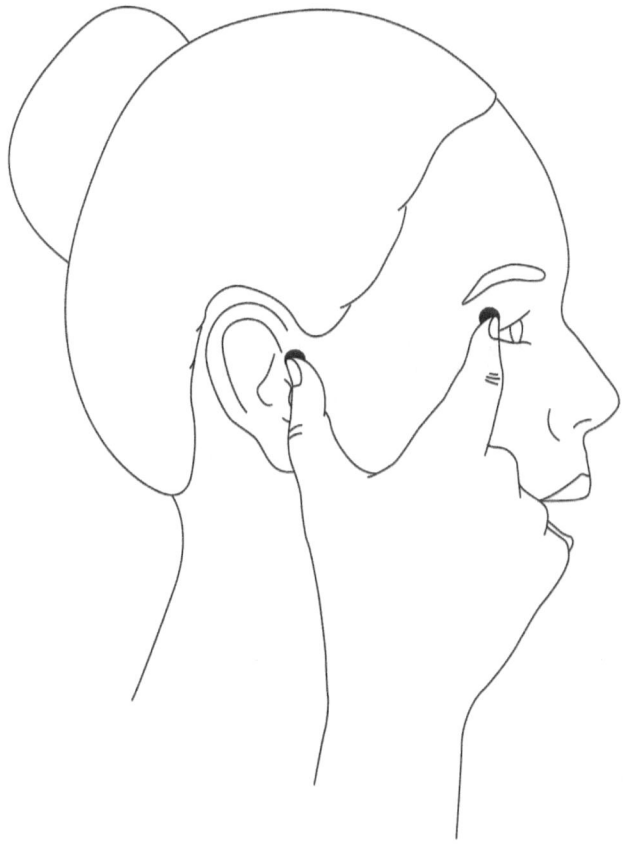

Group 5-A

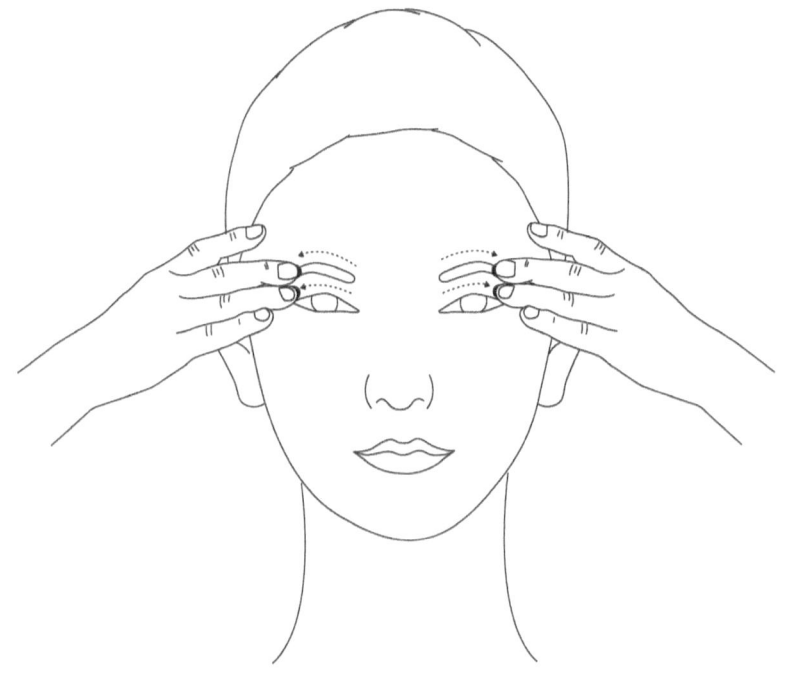

Group 5-B

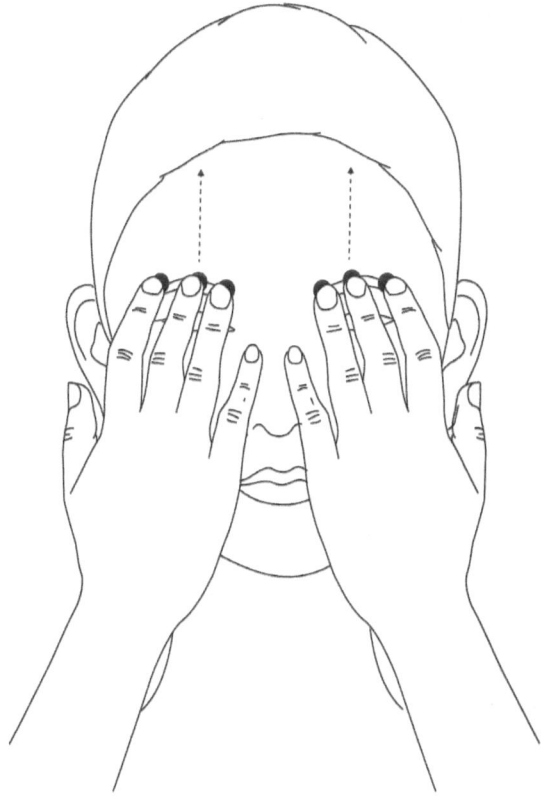

Group 5-C

Group 6

Index fingers press into upper sides[16] (lachrymal gland) of eyes, SJ20[17] with thumbs press into SJ22[18]. Afterwards middle fingers replace index fingers while thumbs move behind ears to SJ19[19].

LACHRYMAL GLAND: ¼ anterior on the upper lid from the end of eye

SJ22: approximately 0.5 cun anterior to the upper border of the root of the ear, in a slight depression on the posterior of the hairline of the temple

SJ20: directly above the ear apex, within the hairline

SJ19: posterior to the ear, at the junction of the upper and middle third of the curve formed by SJ17 and SJ20 behind the helix

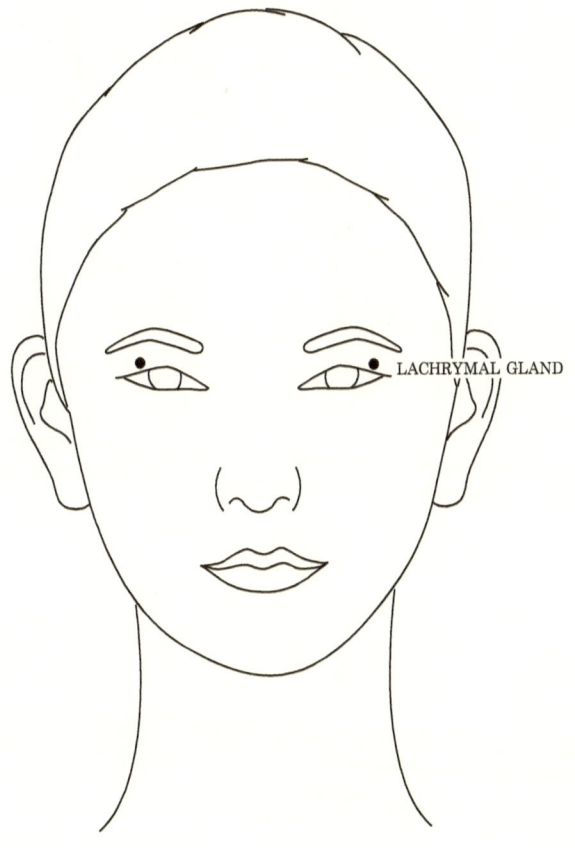

LACHRYMAL GLAND

Group 6

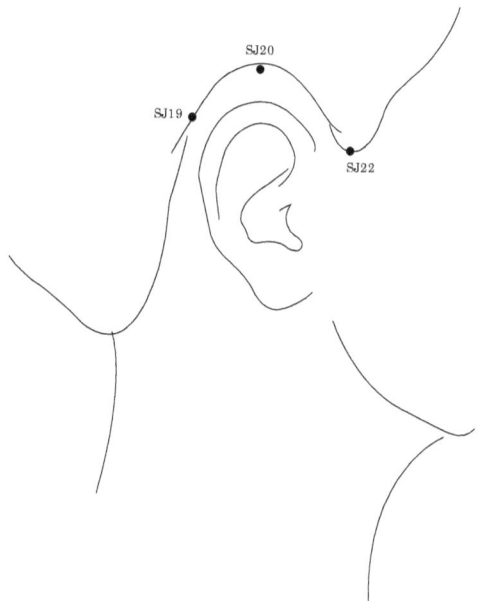

Group 6

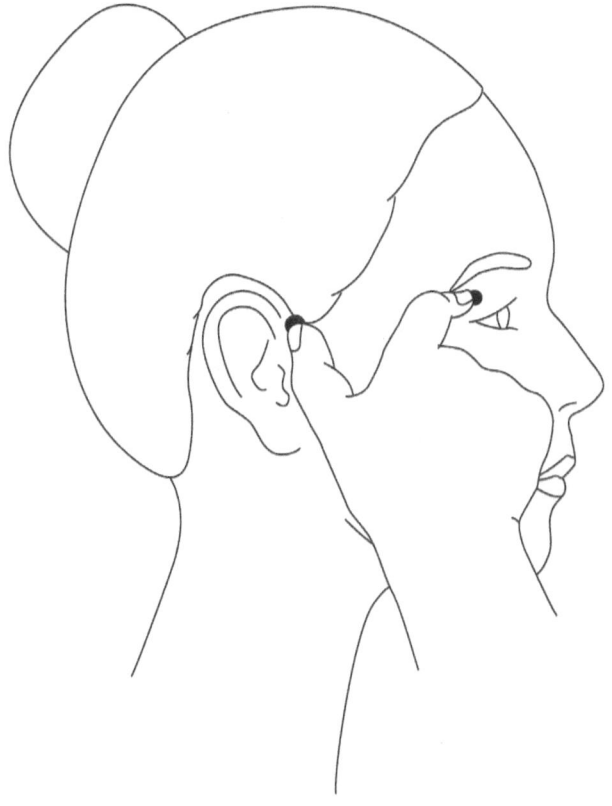

Group 6-A SJ22

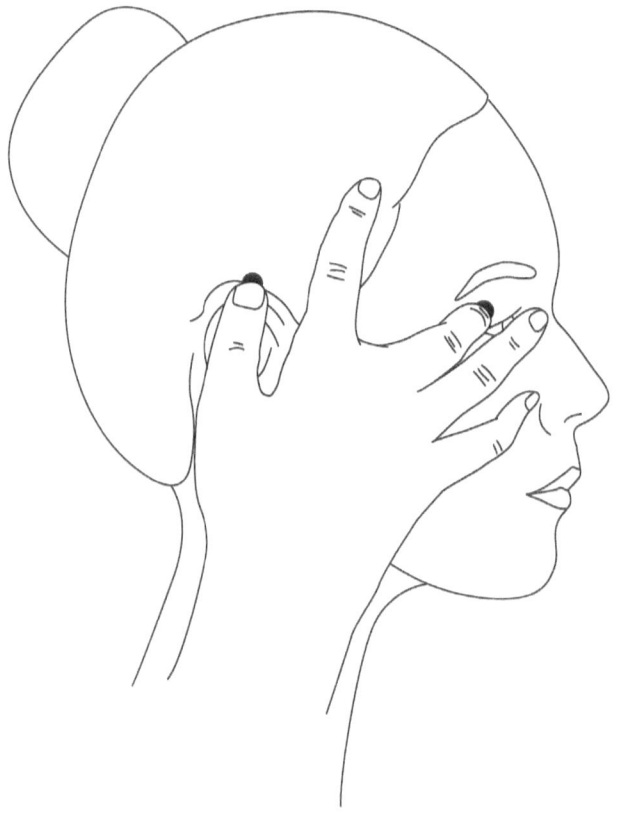

Group 6-A SJ20

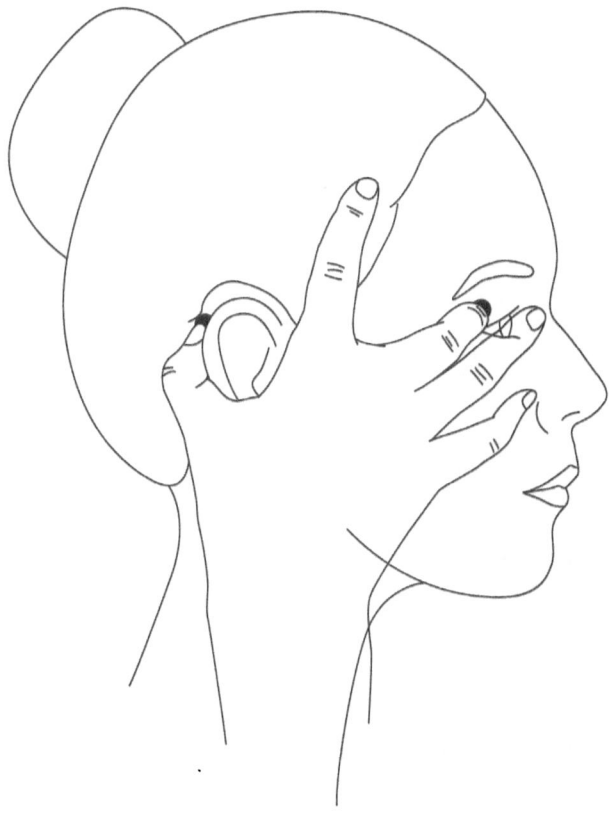

Group 6-A SJ19

Group 7

A. Index fingers press at the point of Taiyang as thumbs press at SJ 18[20] and SJ 17[21] in order.

B. Third fingers press at Taiyang[22] as press thumbs at LI 18[23], ST9[24] and SI 17[25] in order.

SJ18:   in the center of the mastoid process, at the junction of the middle and lower third of the curve formed by SJ17 and SJ 20 posterior to the helix

SJ17:   posterior to the lobule of the ear, in the depression between the mandible and mastoid process

TAI YANG: in the depression about 1 cun posterior to the midpoint between the lateral end of the eyebrow and the outer canthus

- This means greater yang, in another word, sun. This is very important point, however this doesn't belong to regular meridian, but extra point.

LI 18:   on the lateral side of the neck, level with the tip of the Adam's apple, between the sternal head and clavicular head of muscle

ST9:   level with the tip of the Adam's apple, where the pulsation of the common carotid artery is palpable on the anterior border of muscle sternocleidomastoiddeus (SCM)

SI17:   posterior to the angle of the mandible, in the depression on the anterior border of muscle sternocleidomastoiddeus

Please do the following.

When you do Group 6 and 7 on next day, press inner border line of the ear. This is not normal acupuncture points, but very effective.

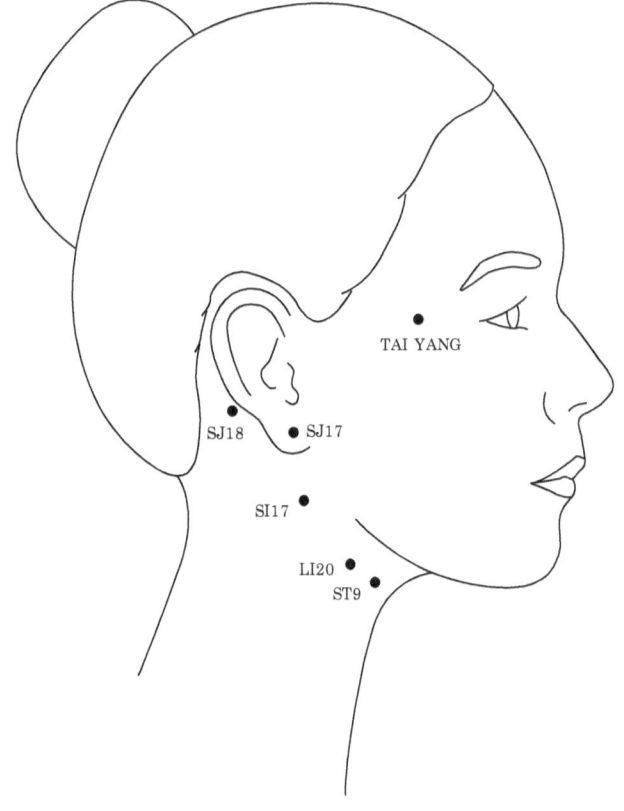

TAI YANG

SJ18

SJ17

SI17

LI20

ST9

Group 7

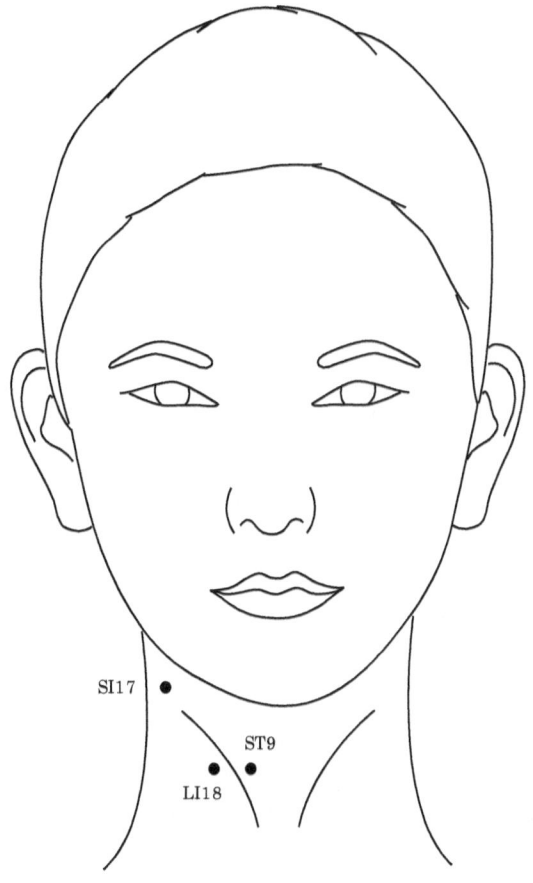

Group 7

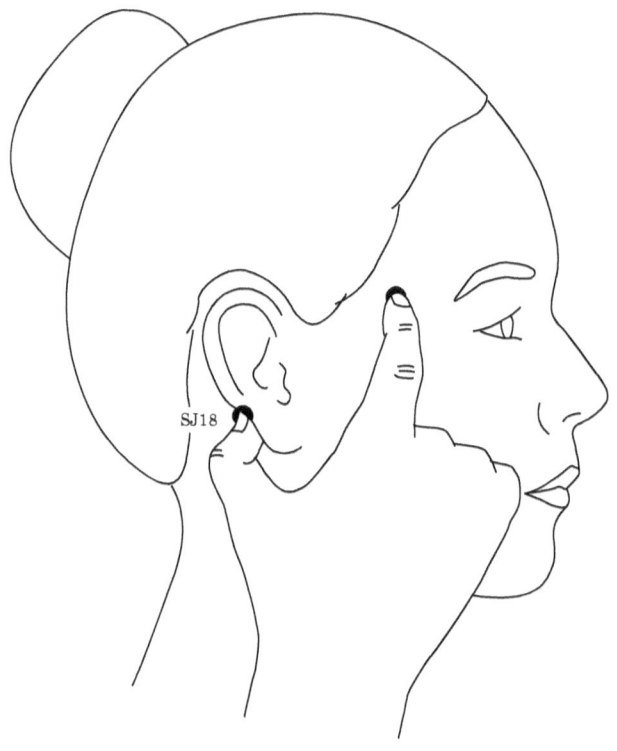

Group 7-A SJ18

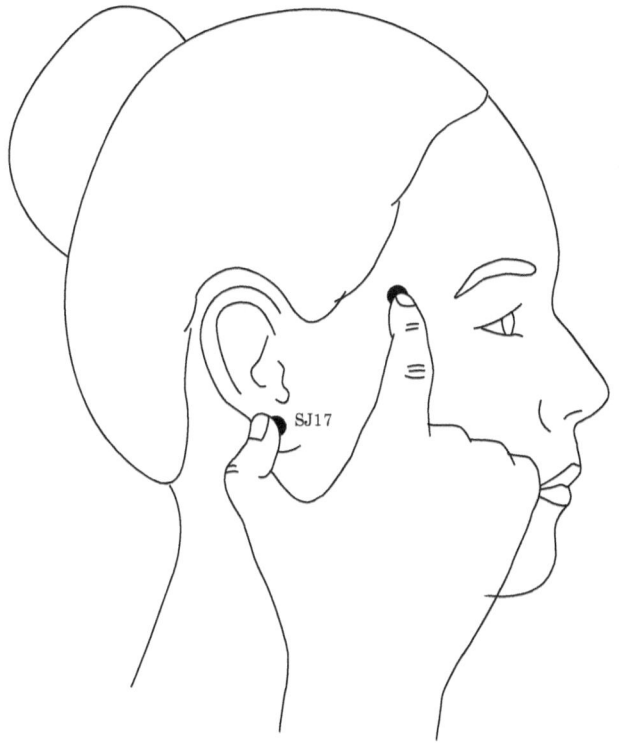

SJ17

Group 7-A SI17

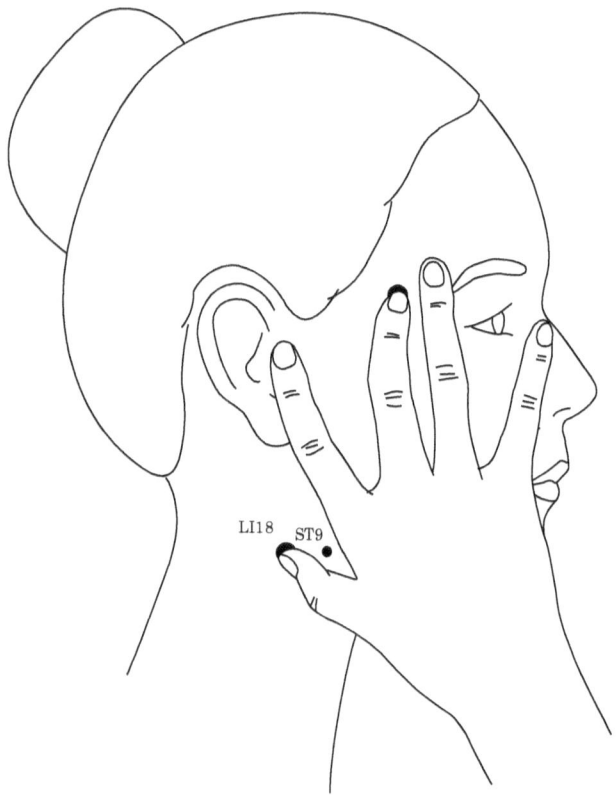

Group 7-B

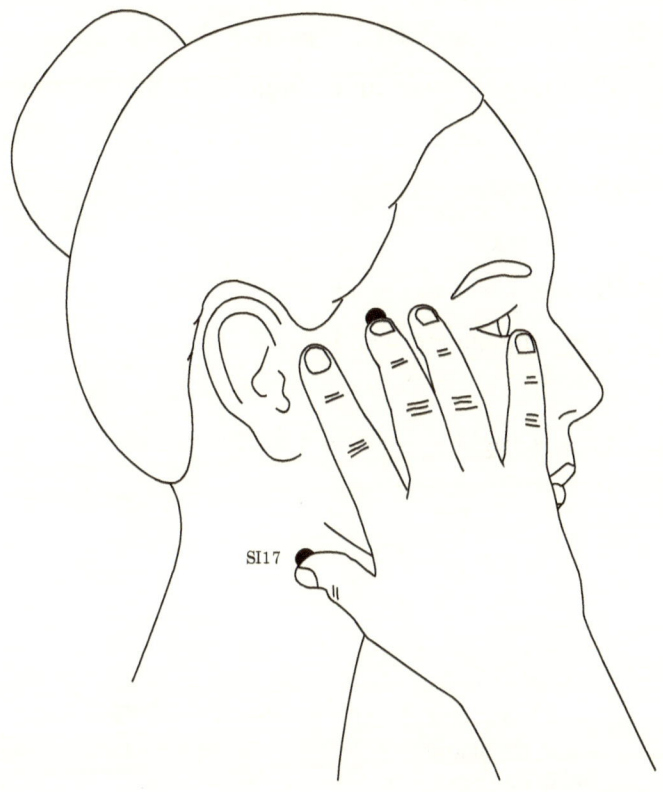

Group 7-C

Group 8

A, All fingers press into sides of head while thumbs press behind head. All fingers press on ST8[26], GB4[27], GB5[28], GB6[29], and GB7[30] as the thumbs press on GB8[31] or GB9[32]. Press index finger on GB7 and pinky finger on ST8 as it is not possible to press 5 points with four fingers.

B. Thumbs press under ears, GB12[33] as other finger tips press into side of head above ears.

C. Thumbs slightly reposition further behind.

ST 8:   at the corner of the forehead

GB4:   within the hairline of the temporal region at the junction of the upper ¼ and lower ¾ of the distance between ST8 and GB7

GB5:   within the hairline of the temporal region midway of the border line connecting ST8 and GB7

GB6:   within the hairline of the temporal region at the junction of the lower1/4 and upper ¾ distance between ST8 and GB7

GB7:   on the head, at the crossing point of the vertical posterior border of the temple and horizontal line through ear apex

GB8:   superior to the apex of the auricle, 1.5 cun within the hairline

GB9:   directly above the posterior border of the auricle, 2 cun within the hairline, about 0.5 cun posterior GB8

ANMIAN: midpoint between SJ17 and GB20

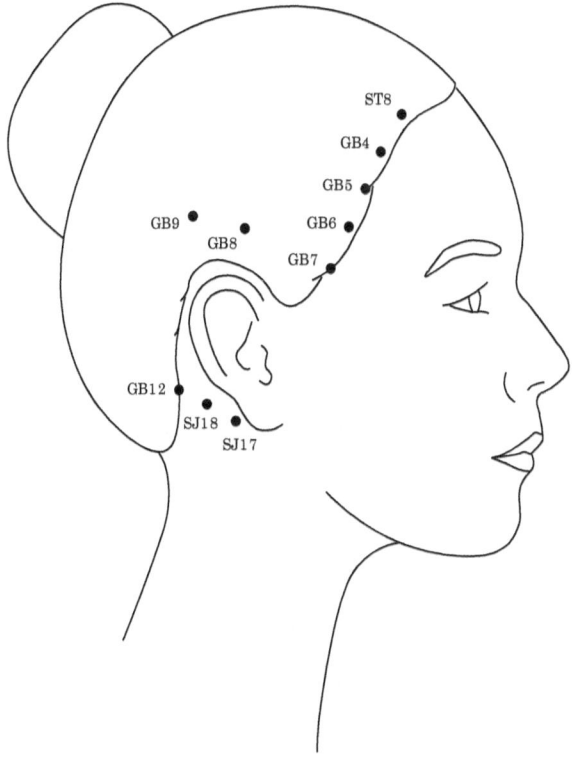

Group 8

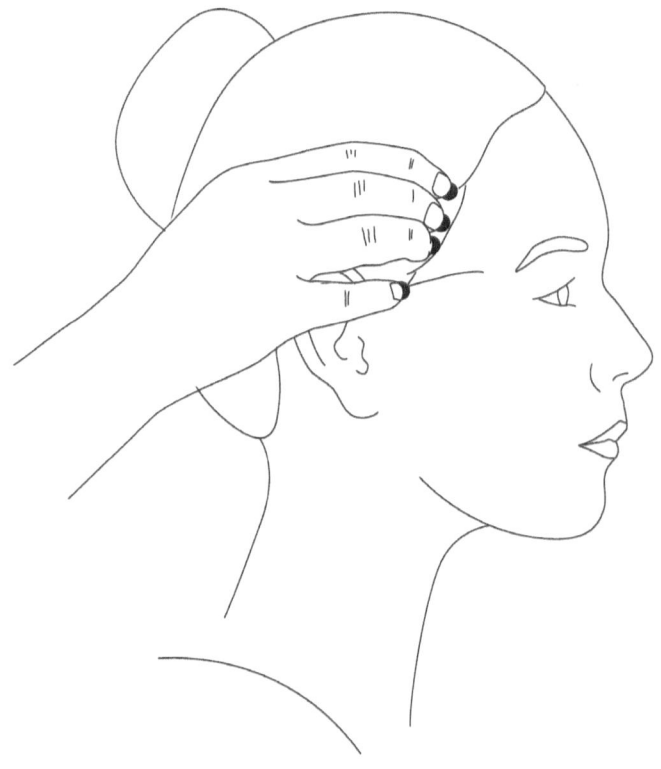

Group 8-A

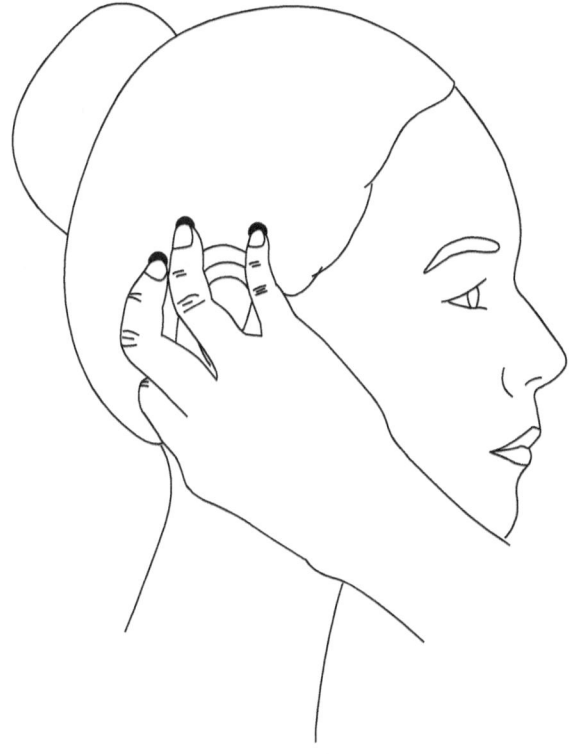

Group 8-B-C

Group 9

A. Forefingers press into sides of nose while thumbs massage lower gum line starting from center to the ears.

B. Index and middle fingers press into sides of nostrils while index fingers of the other hand presses into lower throat area at CV22[34]. This should be alternated with another version where the other hand presses fingers into the sternum for each day.

BITONG: at the highest point of the nasolabial groove

CV22: in the center of the suprasternal fossa

JIACHENGJIANG: 1 cun lateral to CV24

LI20: in the nasolabial groove, at the level of the midpoint of the lateral border of ala nasi

CV16: on the anterior midline, at the level with the fifth intercostal space, on the xiphosternal syhondrosis

CV 17, 18, 19, 20: points between CV16 and CV21

CV21: on the anterior midline, in the center of the sternal manubrium, 1 cun below CV22

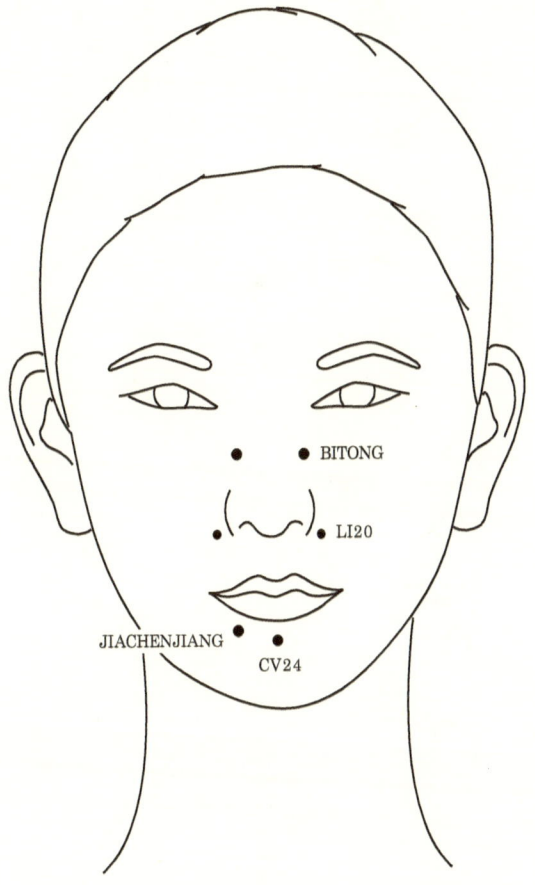

Group 9

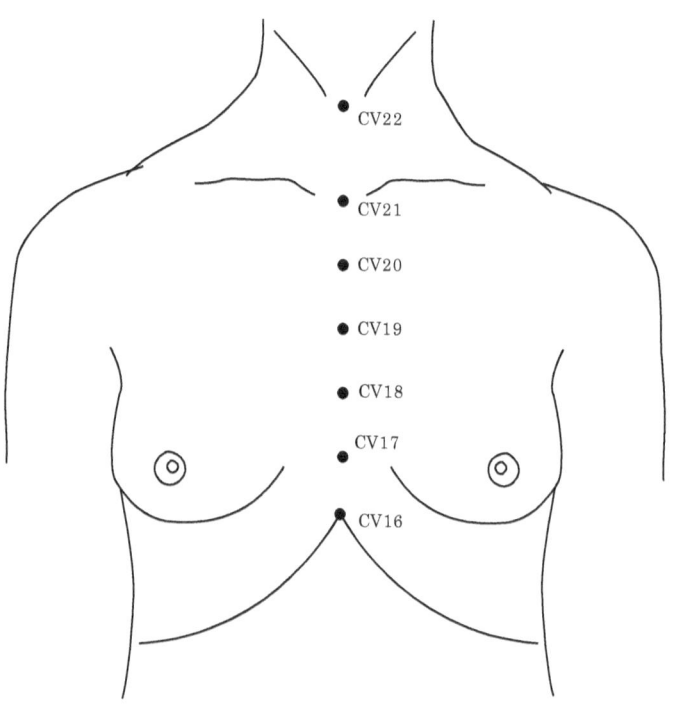

Group 9

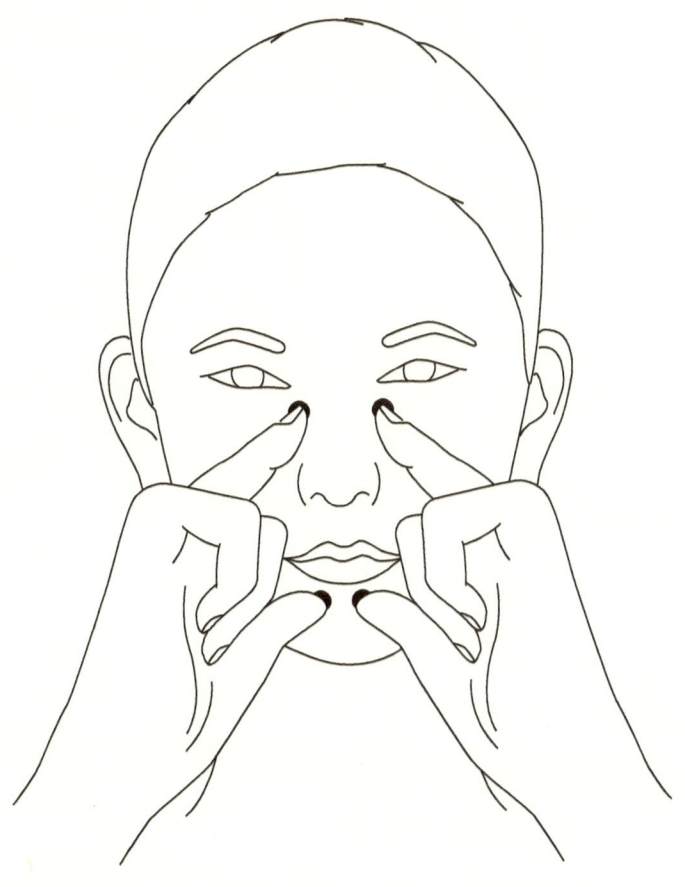

Group 9-A

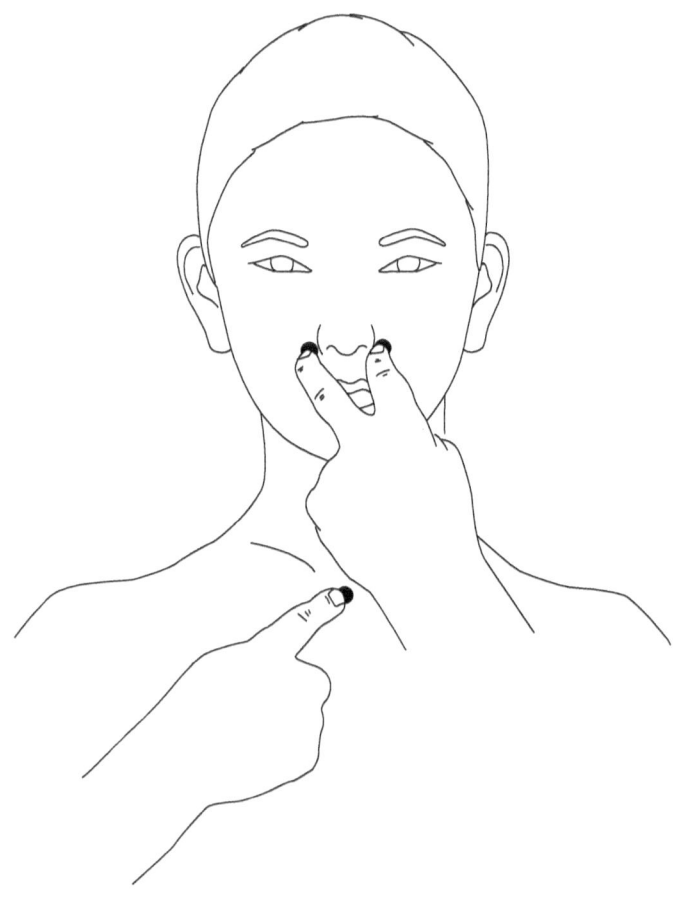

Group 9-B

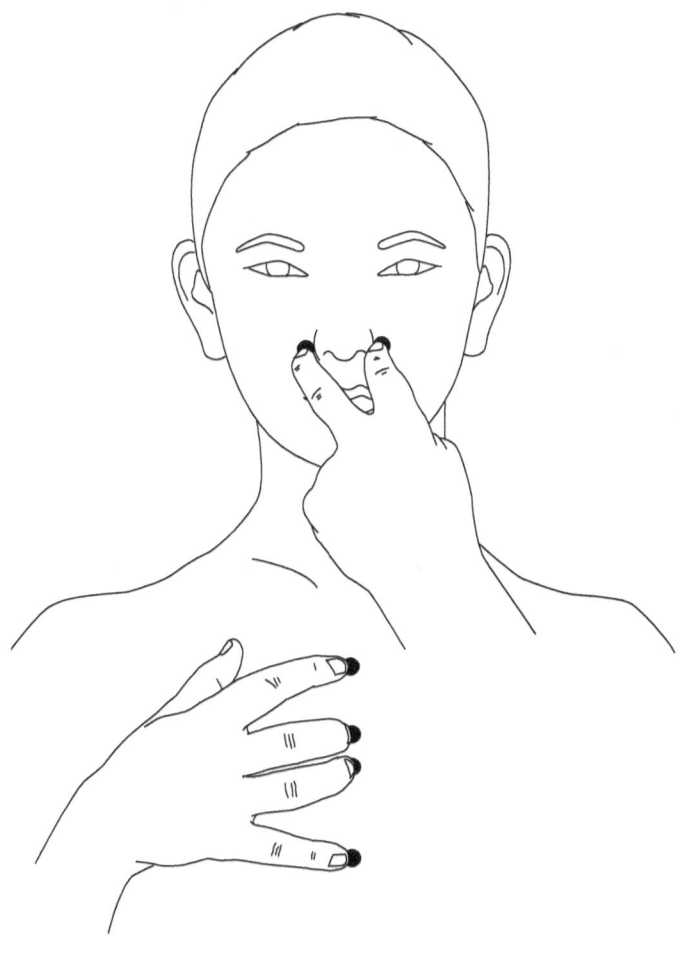

Group 9-C

Deep Breathing

When you do on Group 9, you may experience deep breathing. It depends on how long you have practiced and your inner energy. Many of us never practice at all, even though deep breathing is good for health.

Some experience deep breathing while doing other groups. This depends how long you practice these exercises and how healthy you are. But the level is less than Group 9 generally.

Method of deep breathing

1. Relax the body and breathe in through only the nose while the mouth closes. You continue the abdominal area to be a large balloon.

2. Now hold breathing a moment.

3. Breathe out through the mouth only as the nose should not be used for breathing out. You breathe out until you feel the abdominal area touch the backbone. Breathing out takes twice of time than breathing in.

4. Practice 3-5 times a day.

5. It is better you do more often and longer. You must do at least 3 times per each time. Personally I set up the time as follows: when you get up, while you do Group 9-B, before lunch, before dinner and before bed. I don't forget the time for breathing in this way.

6. When you continue this exercise, you are going to have deep breathing during Group 9-A.

Group 10

Index finger of one hand pull the upper nose area on the inside of eye while the other index finger slides along the lower eye area on the lower eye lid, upper eye lid and lower & upper lids together.

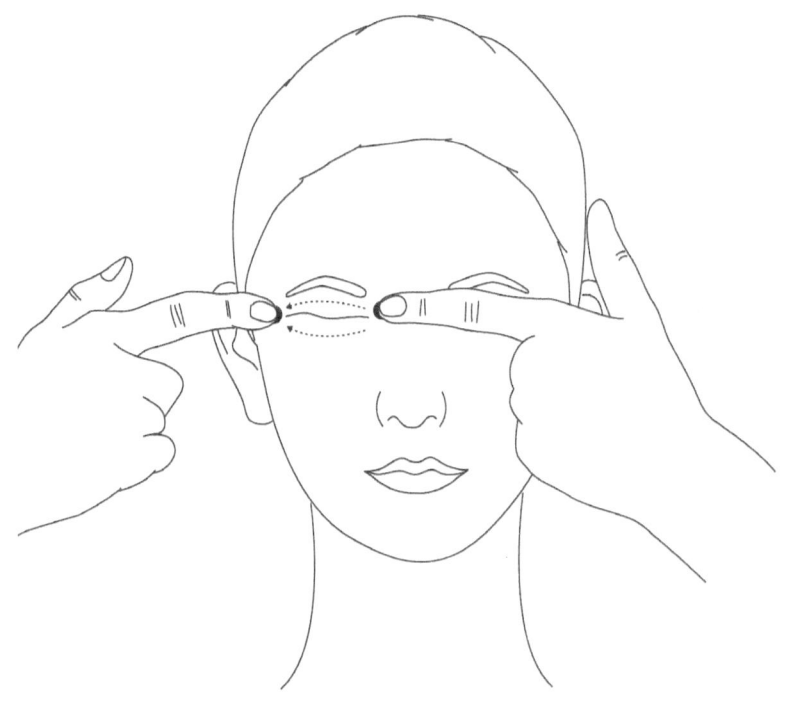

Group 10

Group 11

A. Massage the backbone area at the points; DU14[35], DU13[36], UB11[37], and SJ15[38]. Use the right palm for the right side and left palm for the left side.

B. Stimulate ear lobes with palms.

C. Massage and stimulate the back of the neck.

D. Massage ear grooves with index fingers.

E. Massage GB21[39] alternately with palms. Use the right palm for the left shoulder and the left palm for right shoulder.

- B. In case anyone who has earrings, instead of palms, use thumbs and index fingers and grab and pull out ear lobes.

DU 14: below the spinous process of the seventh cervical vertebrae, approximately at the level of shoulder

DU 13: below the spinous process of the first thoracic vertebra

UB11: 1.5 cun lateral to DU 13, at the level of the lower border of the spinous process of the first thoracic vertebra

SJ 15: at the medial end of the suprascapular fossa

GB21: on the shoulder, directly above the nipple, at the midpoint of the line connecting DU 14 and the acromion, at the highest point of the shoulder

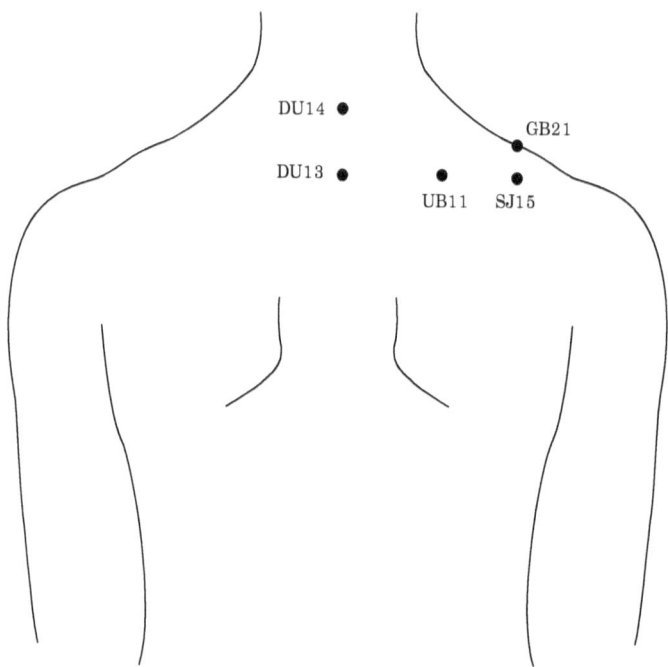

Group 11

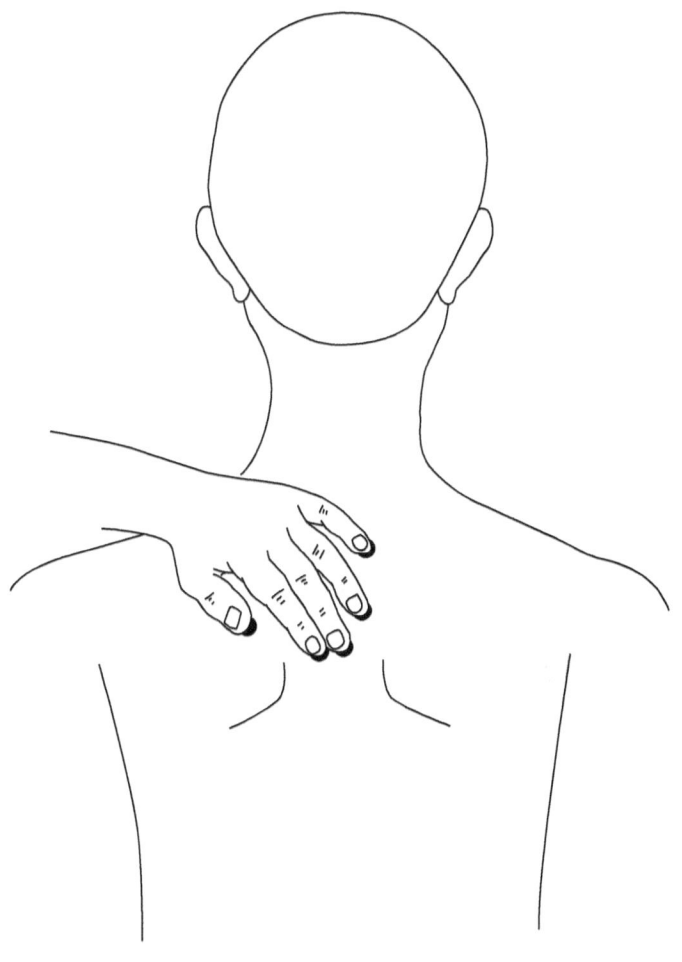

Group 11-A

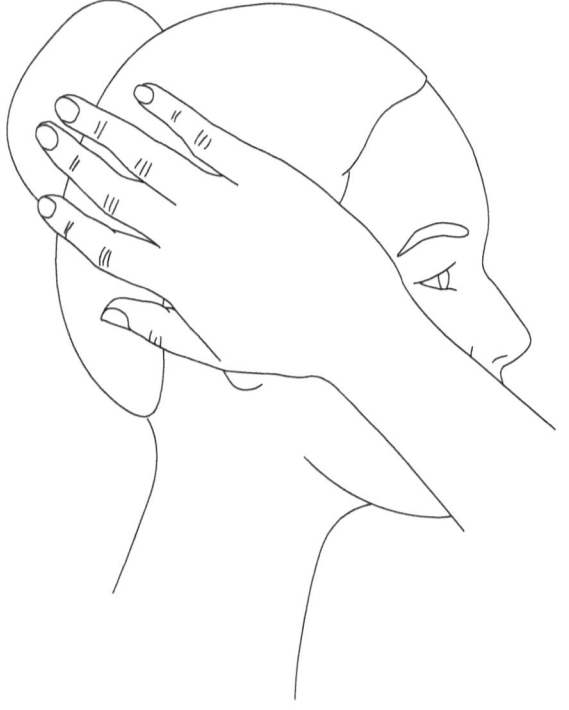

Group 11-B

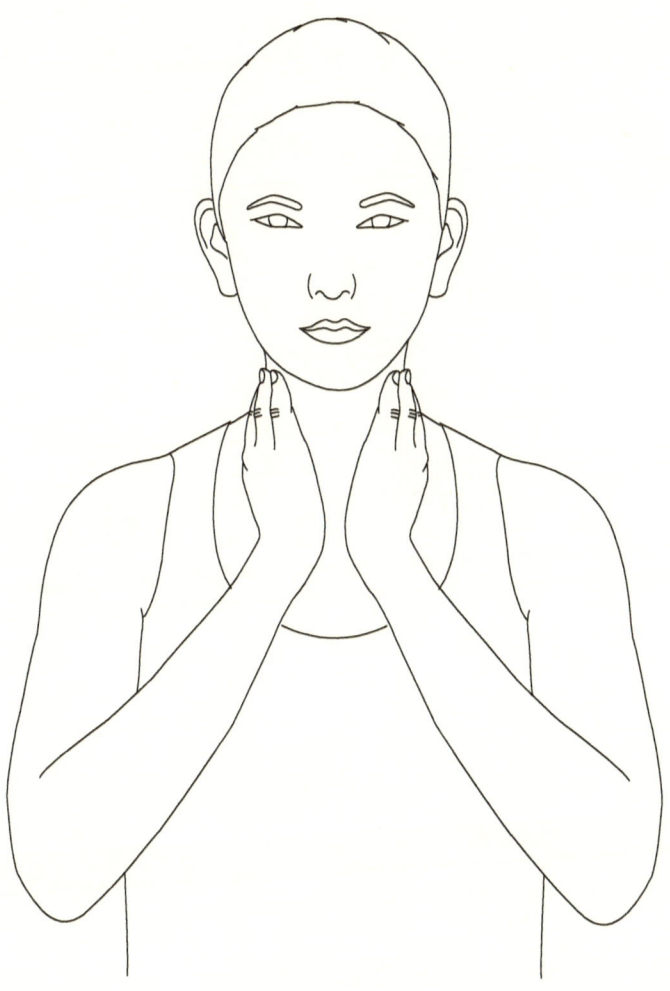

Group 11-C

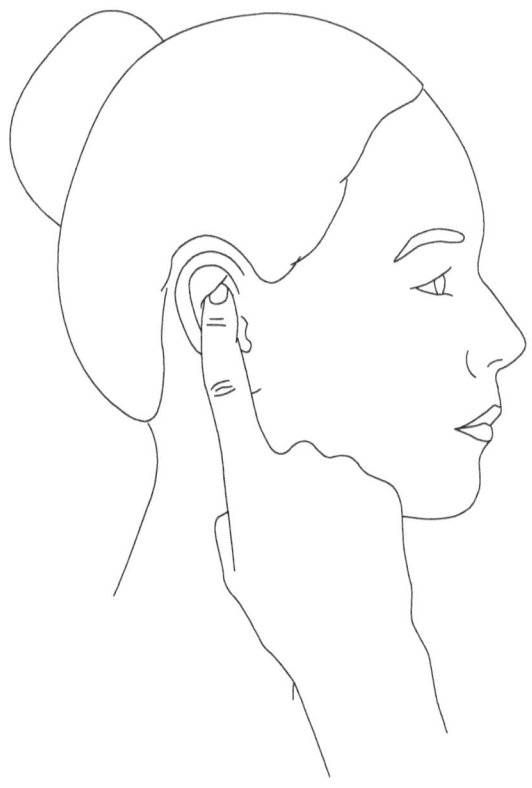

Group 11-D

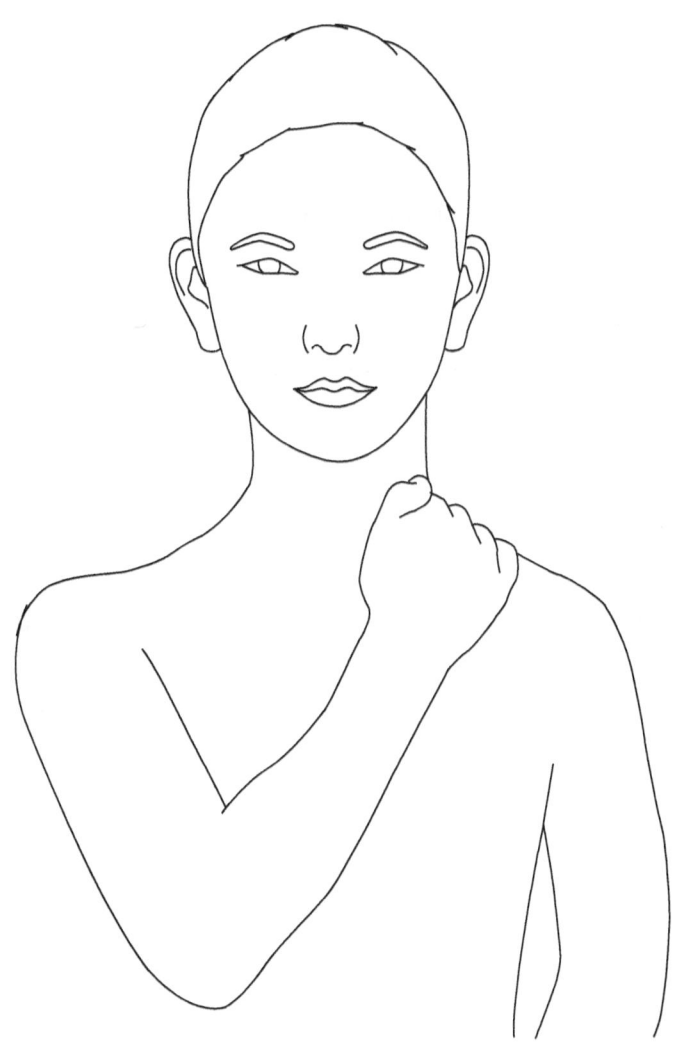

Group 11-E

Tinnitus and Hearing Loss

There are many reasons for tinnitus. Most common are age related hearing loss, Meniere's disease, exposure to loud noise such as working on heavy noise factory or listening loud music, earwax buildup or blockage, stress related etc. Many patients visit an otorhinolaryngologist to check ears and find that there is no specific cause for tinnitus. Some medical doctors suggest alternative treatment such as acupuncture.

According to Traditional Chinese Medicine, kidney function is manifested on ears. This means that the original cause is weakening on kidney function. Some accompany with edema such as acute and chronic nephritic syndrome, congestive heart failure, hepatocirrhosis, endocrine disorders, malnutrition, taking medicine such as prednisone, estrogen and insulin etc. Some accompany with seminal emission such as Prostatitis or neurosis, and impotence and enuresis, urinary dribbling, urinary frequency, incontinence of urine and nocturia. Some complain lower back pain. As you understand, all organs' function is interrelated. Kidney is not working alone.

Tinnitus from kidney dysfunction is that noise stops once in a while, louder noise when tired, noise reduced when pressing ear and dizziness accompanied.

Some are caused by liver hyperactivity, we call liver yang rising. Meniere's disease could belong to liver dysfunction. I don't mention all related symptoms with liver as it is too long. Tinnitus related with liver is that noise is constant without stopping.

Another main cause is from neurotic disease (this is what I name). There is no specific reason. Patients hear sound of wind, whistle blows or the chirp of a cicada. Some complain nervous prostration, hysteria, depression, anxiety and fretfulness. Some accompany with headache, dizziness and insomnia etc.

If tinnitus is less than 2 years, the success rate is high. If more than 5 years, the success rate is very low. As soon as anyone notices any abnormal symptom, we highly recommend seeing professionals right away. Even though you try the following or the sound keeps coming back, you must see the acupuncturist.

One patient who lives at Long Island loves to go to sea with his boat. His tinnitus let him quit the job as the sound was too loud and he couldn't sleep well at all. As the ear sound is similar with sea wave, he couldn't notice while he enjoys fishing on his boat. ENT doctor advised him he couldn't help for his tinnitus after all tests were done. Everything was normal. MD told him some kind of devices is being worked. This sounding devise offsets ear sound, so the patient can't hear the Tinnitus sound. In the mean time, the patient paid $4500 for all kinds of examination. When he came to me, I fold the ear and put my one finger to fold and hit the ear drum couple of times with another finger. Middle finger folds ear lube and index finger put over the middle finger and slides down and hits to ear drum. The sound disappeared instantly. He became furious and said this simple technique stooped the sound, but he believed he spent $4500 for nothing.

Group 12

A. Following upwards urinary bladder meridian, fingers press into UB4[40] (pinky finger) to UB7[41] (index finger). Try to make fingers with straight line.

B. Press UB10[42] with index fingers while pressing UB8 with pinky fingers. The ways of fingers are the same as above. UB8 is very good for myopia. Tap with fingers or rub this point.

C. Press GB14[43] with pinky fingers while pressing GB17 with index fingers.

D. Press GB17[44] with pinky fingers while pressing GB20[45] with index fingers.

[UB4:]   0.5 cun directly above the midpoint of the anterior hairline and 1.5 cun lateral to the midline, at the junction of the medial third and lateral two-thirds of the distance from DU4 to ST8

[UB 5, 6, 7, 8, 9:]   points between UB4 and UB10

[UB10:]   1.3 cun lateral to the midpoint of the posterior hairline and in the depression on the lateral aspect of muscle traperzius

[GB14:]   On the forehead, directly above the pupil, 1 cun directly above the midpoint of the eyebrow

[GB15:]   on the head, directly above the pupil, 0.5 cun above the anterior hairline, at the midpoint of the line connecting DU24 and ST8

[GB 16, 17, 18, 19:]   points between GB15 and GB20

E. Press fingers along the center line, one hand above from DU15[46] (index finger) to DU19[47] (pinky finger) and one hand behind from DU20[48] (index finger) to DU24[49] (pinky finger).

GB20: in the depression between the upper portion of sternocleidomastoideus and muscle trapizius, on the same level with DU16

DU15: 0.5 cun directly above the midpoint of the posterior hairline, in the depression below the spinous process of the first cervical vertebra

DU16, 17, 18, 19: points between DU15 and DU20

DU20: on the midline of the head, 5 cun directly above the midpoint of the anterior hairline, approximately on the midpoint of the line connecting the apexes of both ears

DU 21, 22, 23: points between DU20 and DU24

DU24: 0.5 cun directly above the midpoint of the anterior hairline

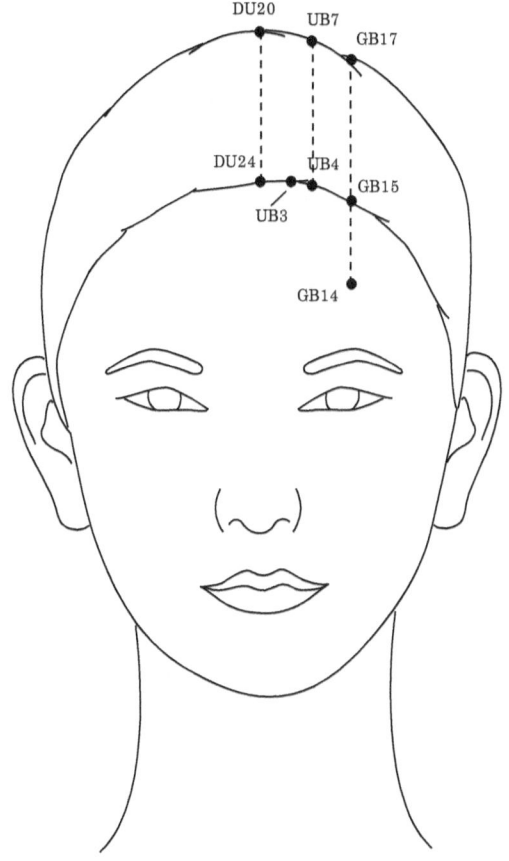

Group 12

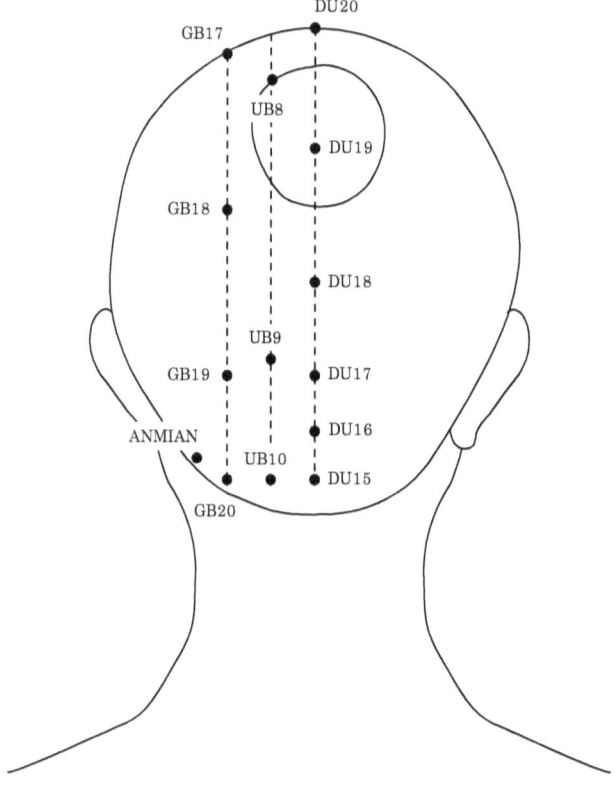

Group 12

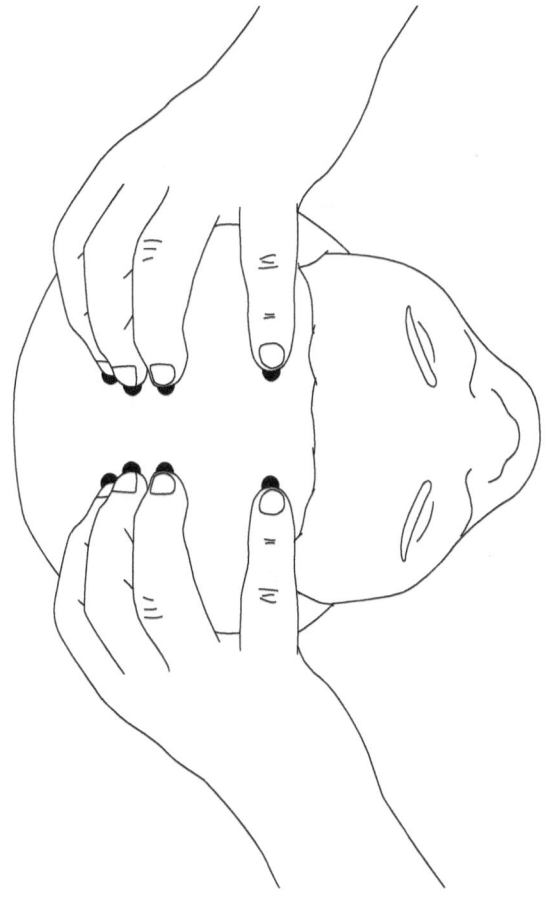

Group 12-A

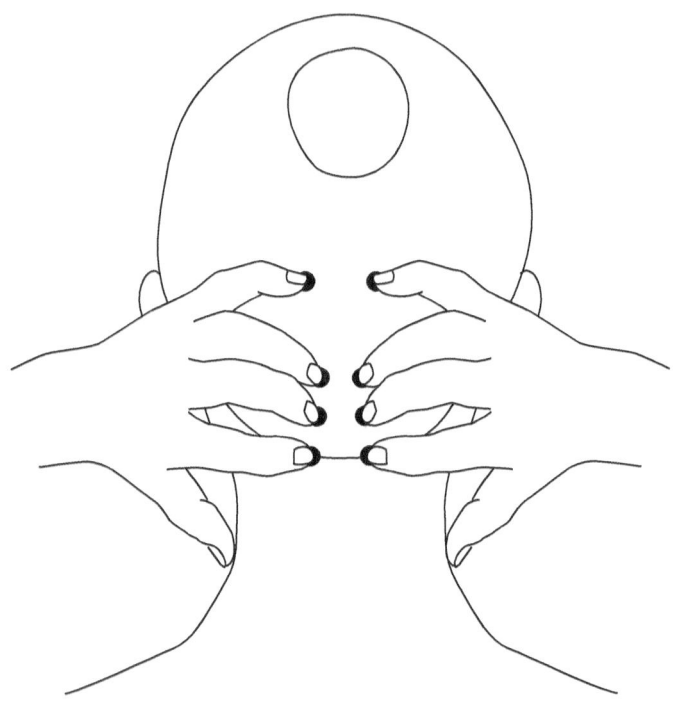

Group 12-B

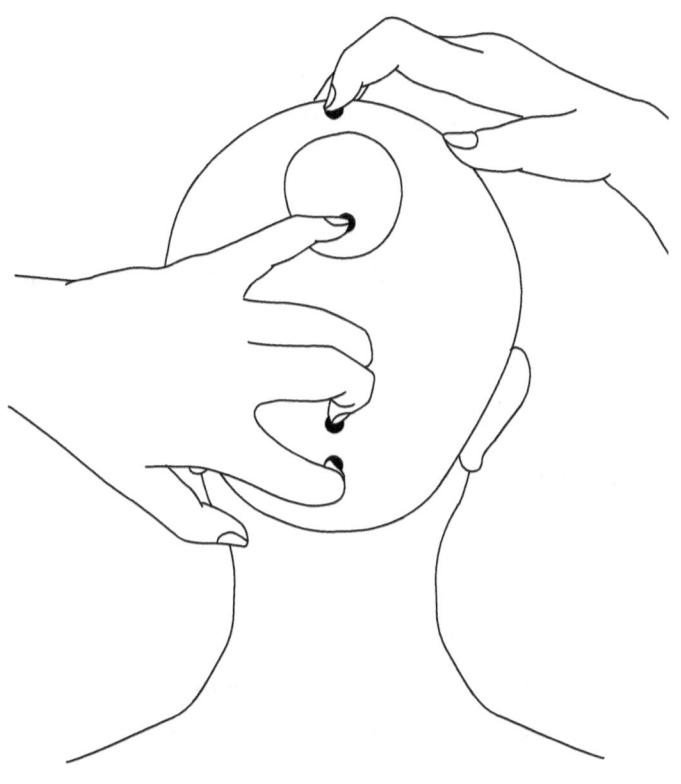

Group 12-C, D, E

Gum massages not covered Group 3 and 9

1. Use a toothbrush and dental floss for gum massage.

2. Use a water pick. This may be better than toothpicks or dental floss in my opinion

3. Massage upper gum and lower gum which behind teeth with the tip of tongue. Continue the same way for gums in front of teeth. While you do this, saliva will be made and collected. While the mouth closes, try to shoot out saliva between teeth.

Good spots for better vision

- SI 6: dorsal to the head of the ulna. When the palm faces the chest, the point is in the bony cleft on the radial side of the styloid process of the ulna

- LI 4: on the dorsum of the hand between the 1st and 2nd metacarpal bones, approximately in the middle of the 2nd metacarpal bone on the radial side

- GB37: 5 cun directly above the tip of the external malleolus, on the anterior border of the fibula

- LR 3: on the dorsum of the foot, in the depression distal to the junction of the first and second metatarsal bones

How to do

Press these points with the tip of fingers or ballpoint pen.

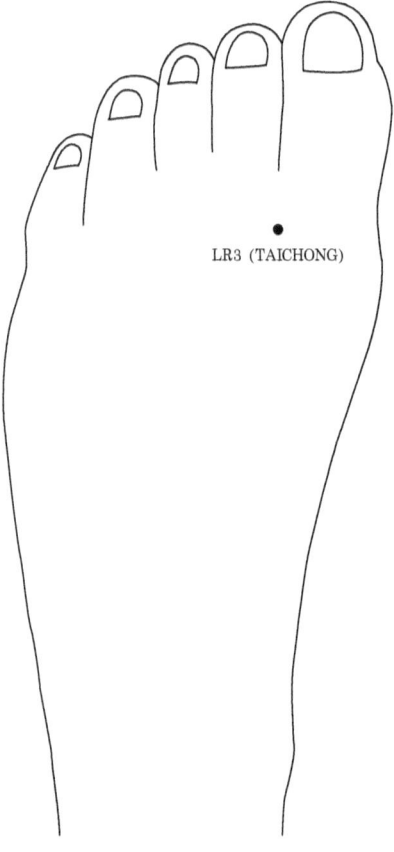

LR3 (TAICHONG)

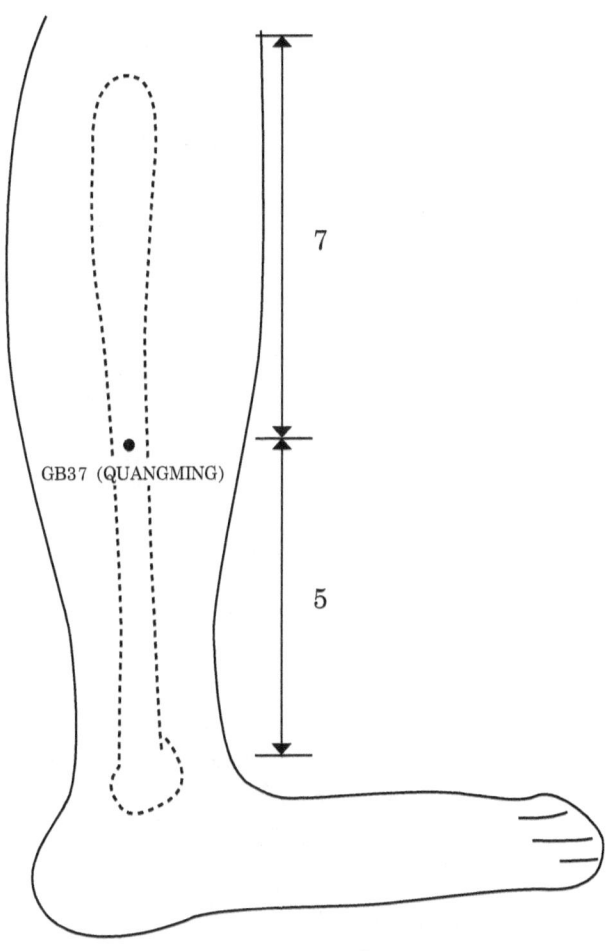

GB37 (QUANGMING)

7

5

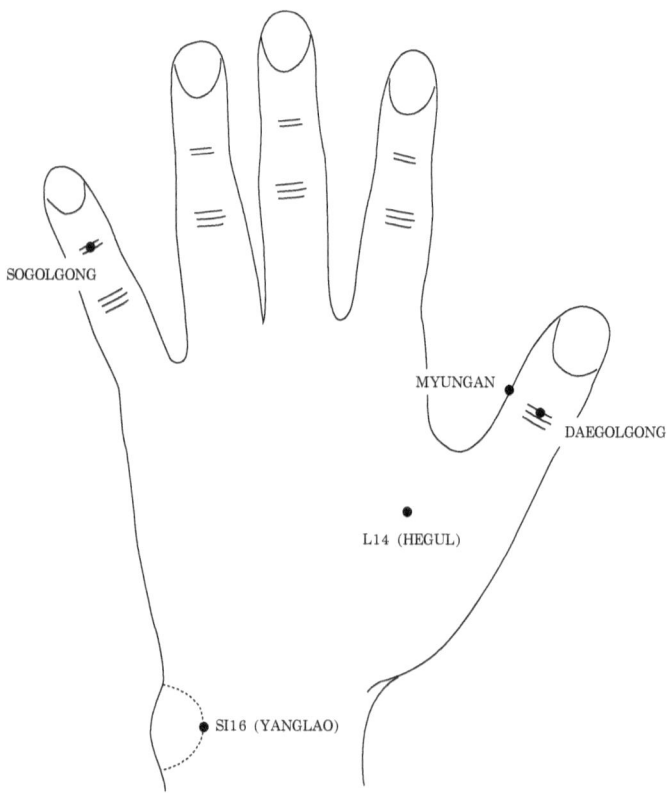

SOGOLGONG

MYUNGAN

DAEGOLGONG

L14 (HEGUL)

SI16 (YANGLAO)

Foods good for eyes

1. Jue Ming Zi: Sweet, bitter and slightly cold, it is also moist in nature. It enters the liver channel to clear heat, drain fire and brighten eyes for eye problems due to wind heat or liver fire blazing up. It also enters large intestine channel to moisten dryness, and unblock the obstruction of bowel movements. (quoted from Materia Medica).

   I also suggest that if liver is excessive, use this tea as it is, but if liver is deficient, use roasted one.

2. Carrot: This is one of vegetables that contain vitamin A helping night blindness. Vitamin A also helps the surface of the eye, mucous membranes and skin be effective barriers to bacteria and viruses, reducing the risk of eye infection, respiratory problems and other infectious diseases.

3. Blueberries: helps to protect and strengthen the vision and to increase macular pigmentation in the eyes.

4. Salmon: Salmon is rich in DHA, which provides structural support to cell membranes and is recommended for dry eyes, treatment for macular degeneration and sight maintenance. Mackerel and blue-backed fishes are good, too.

5. Eat at least one egg per day, as the yolks are especially helpful for raising blood levels of lutein and zeaxanthin by 25 to 30 percent. These nutrients are particularly beneficial in reducing the risk of cataracts and macular degeneration. Try to stick to eggs from pasture-raised chickens, which produce the most beneficial eggs because their diets are rich in nutrients.

6. Liver of animals: helps to strengthen human body's liver. Liver is very closely related with eyes in acupuncture theory

7. Gou Qi Zi: Evenly tonifies the liver and kidney, augments the essence and blood. It is primarily used for liver and kidney insufficiency, or deficiency of both the essence and blood. It also nourishes liver and enhances visual acuity. This is good with blurry vision and decreased visual acuity. Di Huang, Ju Hua and shan zhu yu can be added for better results. (Materia Medica)

How to make Saline solution

Eye doctors recommend artificial tears. I believe saline solution is better with my experience. I don't like to use chemicals into my body as much as possible. Looking for from nature is better than chemicals. Artificial tears contain preservative. Do you think preservative is good for your body? Some contains steroids. I hope you understand side effects for long term use.

The way to make is using distilled water and bamboo salt. Add one spoon of bamboo salt into one gallon of distilled water and mix well. Pour into another bottle through coffee filter. This procedure may eliminate any left over bamboo peels. Keep this saline solution in the dark and cool place. When you need, pour into 16 ounce bottle for gargling. Prepare a small bottle like original bottle for artificial tears. When any kind of small bottle for eyes is used, a suction tool is required.

When you get up, try gargling with saline solution. Even though you can drink, this is used for just cleaning the mouth. You feel instant awakening. You put saline solution into eyes. All sleepiness will be gone.

I read an article that one parent couldn't wake their child up for school. The child missed the school many times. The authority fined parents not to send students for school. If this family knows this idea, the parent may put saline solution into his eyes and the child may get up for school right away.

Why is saline solution used instead of other salts?
When a fetus is inside wombs, it grows in amniotic fluid. Amniotic fluid cleans and purifies fetus' urine and feces. When 9 months passes after the pregnancy, the intensity of amniotic fluid is similar with sea water. What is the content of amniotic water? Do you think sea water consists of only NaCl? The answer should be NO. This means our body is familiar with salt before we born.

Most tables have salt which costs less. This salt provides salty taste, but contains only NaCl. There are no other minerals. Let us review NaCl how it works in the body.

NaCl works on sympathetic nerve system. What about parasympathetic nerve? Potassium works on here. There is unbalance between NaCl and potassium if you use just cheap salts. All other minerals are none on cheap salts. We know all other minerals are required for our body. Therefore you understand the body needs balanced in minerals, which is sea salt.

Here is another issue to discuss. All polluted materials which are used by human beings are flowed into sea eventually. Real salts are produced from salt fields. Even though salts are produced from sea farms, we have to worry about pollution. In order to eliminate polluted materials from sea salts, we'd better use with bamboo salts which are made by special procedures. The problem is the bamboo salts are very expensive depending on how many times this salt is processed. Some are processed by 9 times.

Due to expensive prices, I personally use 2 times processed one whose PH number is 7.2. This number is identical with our body. We add this bamboo salts for our cooking and even for home made juices.

AN OPTION FOR YOU

I began this hoping my gray hair to black. But it has not happened yet. I do believe the idea is going to work on the following steps, but no result yet on hair color change. That's why I am reluctant to reveal this idea now, so make an option.

I prepare saline water into the basin before the bowel movement in the morning. The water in the basin must hot. The water amount depends on the basin. The water depth must be enough to sink feet up to the Achilles' tendon. The amount of salt is about 50g and amount water is 1 gallon or a little more.

The reason to use hot water is to raise energy up. This would make heavy one downward.

The salt used here must be sea salt. The reason to use the salt is as the body has 0.9% of salt. The density of salt in this basin is much higher than in the body. Therefore osmosis will occur between the body and saline water. We may expect effete mater coming down which may be heavy and good energy bringing up which may be light. Effete matter may come out through the sole of the feet by osmosis. These waste materials are collected and accumulated under the sole. When the time is passed by, whole skin comes off from sole. I had this experiences three times. The thickness was 2-3mm. I didn't analyze the contents of peeling, but sure lots of toxics.

I wash the face with this water. When you begin, I want you use the light density of saline water. If the density is too strong, you feel the burning sensation on the face. If this happens, wash the face with regular water right away.

The face skin is very sensitive. The face skin reflects of conditions of body organs. For example, if the face skin is dry, this means the rising heat consumes moisture making dry. Many believe dry skin is caused by ultraviolet rays. This is true, but not always.

Most cases are from organ dysfunction. Even though removing rising heat is the right method, most just use moisturizer only. This helps, but not the right method for me. Therefore the best is providing proper blood circulation by removing heat from related organs. Acupuncture and herb treatments must be the basic, but saline water may be one method, too.

I also wash my hairs. I believe nutrition may reach to the head making my gray hair to black theoretically, but this doesn't happen yet. What I experience was some sores on head. When I touch sores, there were boils which color was yellow. When I stripped off boils, ooze came out from a sore. It became into normal head skin. These happened usually on the top part of the head. After a few years passed, boils grow on the sides and back area.

When you wash the head, it is better to leave the saline water for 2-3 minutes. While I leave the saline water on my head, I do tooth brushing to save time. I also suggest you this exercise during tooth brushing. Man holds testicles lightly and rubs and presses with fingers and palm. In the beginning you may feel the pain. The pain will be less when the time passes by. Female massages on breasts.

Please note this saline water may prevent loss of hairs and dandruff.

ABOUT THE AUTHOR

The author pursues the practical thing than a theory.

Economy is to study how to be rich in a short sentence. If so, the richest man in theory must be a professor in economics. However most professors do live comfortably, but they are not the richest person.

Mr. Anthony Robinson said that if you want to be a best in a certain field find the best and copy him. While I study in the TCM School, I try to find a best acupuncturist. It had taken a year to find a true master to me. I bought his books and seminar materials and studied his books. There are a few information that I have not learned in the school. This idea makes me one of Korean 4 needle specialists.

I could develop some unique approaches that guarantee eczema treatment and acne to be healed within one month. If I don't treat within a month, I treat next month on me. If I still don't treat as promised, I will return the money paid. Is there any more practical way than this?

The books I write would be practical one. Once anyone used it, so easy to follow.